MY MEDICAL SCHOOL

Other titles in this series (General Editor: Dannie Abse)

MY OXFORD

MY CAMBRIDGE

MY LSE

MY DRAMA SCHOOL

Forthcoming :

MY ART SCHOOL

MY MUSIC SCHOOL

MY MILITARY ACADEMY

MY MEDICAL SCHOOL

DANNIE ABSE   MARTIN BAX   ELLIA BERSTOCK
SIR DERRICK DUNLOP   LESLEY ISENBERG
EDWARD LOWBURY   MICHAEL O'DONNELL
LORD PLATT   WILLIAM SARGANT
SHEILA SHERLOCK   JOHN STONE
MIRIAM STOPPARD   PATRICK TREVOR-ROPER

Edited and introduced by
DANNIE ABSE

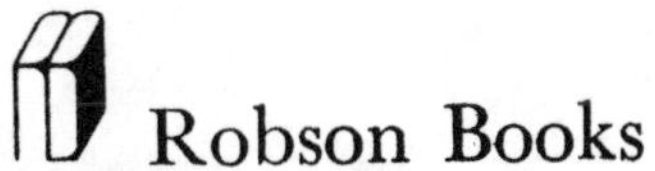

Robson Books

FIRST PUBLISHED IN GREAT BRITAIN IN 1978
BY ROBSON BOOKS LTD., 28 POLAND STREET,
LONDON W1V 3DB. COPYRIGHT © 1978 ROBSON
BOOKS

My medical school
    1. Medical students—Great Britain
    I. Abse, Dannie
    610′.7′1141   R772

    ISBN 0–86051–030–1

Printed in Great Britain by R. J. Acford Ltd., Chichester,
Sussex

CONTENTS

INTRODUCTION

It is hoped that these autobiographical essays will allow the reader genuine amusement; but they are also offered as social documents. Inevitably, since the contributors to this volume range from the elderly to the young (most were trained at different medical schools), testimony is given of the way medical education has progressed over a sixty-year period. Certain educational methods seem not to have changed a jot and are common to all centres—even the conning of medical students into stupidly tasting urine in order to learn an important observational lesson is apparently practised in more than one medical school, and the dramatic, if gentle, reduction of the medical student by his doctor-superior is often accomplished with a delightful originality.

For instance, lately, medical students at the University of California in Los Angeles were asked whether a certain lady should have had her pregnancy terminated given her medical history. The doctor-superior said, 'Her husband had had syphilis, she herself had tuberculosis. They already had four children—the first blind, the second died, the third was deaf and dumb, and the fourth had tuberculosis. So here she was, pregnant again, with her fifth child, and she and her husband both were willing to have had an abortion. So what would you guys have advised?' Almost all the students voted for the pregnancy to be terminated. They were offered congratulations and told that, OK they had just murdered Beethoven! When challenged about the accuracy of Beethoven's medical history, the doctor-superior said that the anecdote was one way of catching class attention.

Doubtless what have proved to be effective techniques and aids in the education of the medical students of yesterday and today will be of use tomorrow. The reader may well decide from these memoirs that there are more similarities than differences in the medical student's general experience despite the time and place of education. Lord Platt's educational exposure at Sheffield during the First World War may have been more dangerous, because of contagious disease, than Dr Isenberg's recent, vivid trials at Cardiff, but the similarities are pronounced—even their reactions sometimes echo each other. 'I hated dissecting the face of a corpse,' writes Lord Platt. 'I hated dissection,' declares Lesley Isenberg. 'Compare and contrast,' growls the teeth-bared solemn examiner.

To the general public the doctor remains a much respected and respectable figure, despite a healthy modern irreverence. Come to think of it, that irreverence is hardly modern. Molière's views of doctors were not solitary. 'I intend to keep to physick all my life,' Molière made his doctor wickedly say, 'I find it is the best trade of all because whether we do good or whether we do harm, we are always paid at the same rate. In short, what is good about this profession is that there is among the dead an honesty and a discretion unexcelled in the world. You never see them complain of the doctor who killed them.' Molière's irreverence had not only a future but a long history. It was Pliny who complained that the Greek physician was the only citizen who could kill another with sovereign impunity.

Some of the doctors who contribute to this volume have their own acid comments to make about old teachers and of the fashionable treatment of their day. Others predictably celebrate their teachers triumphantly and with gratitude—predictably because the history of medicine has many repetitious pages testifying that some of the greatest doctors have also been among the greatest teachers. Hippocrates himself in 400 BC wandered throughout Greece teaching at different medical centres, to leave behind him many pupils who could and did carry on his methods. The Hippocratic Corpus—though nowadays no doctor may read its seventy books—still informs the spirit of modern medicine insofar as it emphasizes the importance of the observation of facts and data, the scepticism of the so-called miraculous, and the hesitating possibility of generalizing from the particular.

Of course there are good teachers and bad ones, good doctors and bad; but for the student of medicine, be he apprentice or qualified physician, there is no such thing as a bad patient. Every patient, in one sense, teaches his physician something about the subject of medicine. If, despite the Molières of this world, the doctor continues to retain a prestigious and reliable reputation, the medical student's image is altogether more awry and dubious. Because of Hollywood, TV medical series, popular books, he is regarded as a wild blundering creature, more interested in the sexual charms of nearby convenient nurses than in the pathology of his victims—that is to say his patients. This book, it must be admitted, does not entirely dispel this robust image. Stories abound here, sometimes shocking as well as hilarious, sometimes sorrowful as well as odd. How could it be otherwise when medical students spend their clinical years in hospitals—in sanctuaries, need it be said, for those who have fallen out from, not always temporarily, 'the splendid procession of Life'?

Doctors cannot fail to be interested in these reminiscences of their colleagues who were trained in one or another of the thirty-three medical schools of the United Kingdom, or indeed in the memoirs of Dr John Stone, a leading American cardiologist, but this book, finally, is intended for the interest and curiosity of the general public—long may they not become patients.

DANNIE ABSE

Lord Platt

Lord Platt was born in London in 1900. He was a medical student at Sheffield University where he qualified MB, ChB in 1921. After serving as a House Physician in Sheffield and London, and spending two years in Pathology, he became Medical Registrar, and later, Physician to the Royal Infirmary, Sheffield. During the Second World War he served as OC Medical Division in hospitals in North Africa and Italy, and later as Consulting Physician of Southern Army, India, with the rank of Brigadier. After the war he became the first whole-time Professor of Medicine in Manchester.

In 1957 he was elected President of the Royal College of Physicians of London, and during his presidency was successful in moving the college from its old inadequate premises in Trafalgar Square to a new building in Regent's Park. He has written 3 books, including his auto-biography Private and Confidential, *and has published many papers in medical journals. He has been a member of the Medical Research Council, and Chairman of its Clinical Research Board. He has honorary degrees of 4 universities and is an honorary member of many medical societies and institutions at home and abroad. He was created a Baronet in 1959 and raised to the Peerage in 1967.*

y medical school was Sheffield. The University, when I first knew it, was only ten years old. The Medical School was a small one, further depleted by the 1914–18 War. There were, I think, only about twelve medical students in my year, and yet Sheffield, then, was perhaps the most advanced medical school in the whole of Great Britain. This statement clearly needs justification.

Medical schools of a rather primitive type, often privately owned, had existed for many years in most provincial cities. In Sheffield from 1828. They were places where students could study anatomy and learn some elementary physiology while being apprenticed to Physicians or Surgeons in hospital or in general practice. The students would then have to pass some external examination of the Society of Apothecaries or of the Royal Colleges or the London MB, BS, which would give them a licence to practise medicine. Towards the end of the nineteenth century the three major seats of higher education in Sheffield, namely, Firth College, the Technical School and the Medical School, having by now greatly improved their standards, amalgamated to form the Sheffield University College which, in 1905, was granted its charter as Sheffield University.

Some of the personalities most deeply concerned in this transition were of course still active ten years later, when I first joined the University, and were among my teachers. Yielding now to autobiographical temptation, I will try to explain how I became a student of Sheffield University. The Platt family derived its name from the Platt district of Manchester in the reign of Edward III, but I was born and brought up in London and my branch of the family had been Londoners for four generations. Being born in 1900 has saved me a great deal of mental arithmetic and I was of course ten years old in 1910 when, owing to a change in the family fortunes, my father and mother decided to set up a co-educational boarding school in Grindleford in the Peak District of Derbyshire. My father, like many I have known whose search for knowledge has not been hampered by a university education, was tremendously well informed. His main interests were in European history, Shakespeare's plays, music, nature study, poetry, architecture and geology. He wrote poetry and music, had visited every cathedral in England and wrote a book on geology. My mother was well advanced in the educational world and at the age of thirty-four was the first woman to become one of Her Majesty's Inspectors of Schools. Her colleagues greatly regretted her marriage in 1897. Whether I regret it depends on my mood-swings. On the whole I think I applaud it.

When I was fifteen I wondered what to do, for I had already passed the matriculation examination which was then the entrance to a university. I did not want to be a teacher. I was no scientist nor was I, like my brother, a natural engineer. Medicine and the Law seemed to be the alternatives and I chose Medicine for two reasons: first because I felt that at the least you would be trying to do some good, whereas I was less certain of the Law in that respect; and secondly because my then current girl-friend (as we would now call her) wanted to marry a doctor. In the event she married someone else long before I qualified. And so, as my parents could not afford to send me to Oxford or Cambridge, my father took me to see Dr Arthur Hall who was then Dean of the Faculty of Medicine in Sheffield University.

Sheffield being a new university with no traditions, my father asked point-blank whether it might not be better for me to go to Edinburgh which had then a medical school of some repute and much tradition. I remember, vividly, Arthur Hall saying, 'There is nothing which Edinburgh can teach him which he cannot better learn in Sheffield.' How right he was I only discovered many years later.

At fifteen I was ill-instructed in Science. Besides, I could not enter as a medical student until I was sixteen, so I spent the year with some further coaching in Latin, which I have never regretted, although its direct relevance to medicine no longer exists. I also attended an elementary course in Physics and Chemistry at Sheffield University, equivalent perhaps to an 'A' level course in a polytechnic college of today. This taught me many things besides Physics and Chemistry. It was an opportunity to grow up and to make the metamorphosis from school to university. It introduced me to students of other Faculties, to young ladies, one of whom I deeply admired, as well as young men.

And so, after this preliminary year, at the age of sixteen, I became a fully-fledged medical student. Our first year was devoted to the three Sciences: Physics, Chemistry and Zoology, and, as it is one of my aims to demonstrate how advanced Sheffield was in relation to other medical schools, I might here point out that Latin had already (in 1915) been deleted as a compulsory subject in matriculation for entrance to the medical course, and Botany had already been discarded as a subject for study for the First MB examination, which came at the end of the first year. (Nowadays many, if not most, students skip the first year altogether, having already achieved adequate standards in their 'A' levels.)

In that first year all our lectures were given by our professors who did not deem it beneath their dignity to take classes for first-year students. The practical work was supervised by members of their staff. For Physics we had W. M. Hicks (1850–1934), in some ways the greatest of them all; the veritable founder of Sheffield University, a wrangler of Cambridge, one of the first students under Clerk Maxwell at the newly opened Cavendish Laboratory; a Fellow and Royal Medallist of the Royal Society whose scientific work, which he continued to his death, was mainly in the mathematical aspects of Physics. One of his sons, Basil Hicks, was killed in that horrible war of 1914–18 which haunted the first years of my student days. The telegram came while he was at lunch in the Refectory. He quietly said 'My turn has come' and left the room. For Chemistry we had William Palmer Wynne (1861–1950), already a Fellow of the Royal Society eight years before he came to Sheffield in 1904. His personal research was in Organic Chemistry, but this was to some extent in abeyance during his Sheffield years because of his untiring devotion to university affairs.

Having coped with the first-year studies under Hicks and Wynne, we turned to Anatomy and Physiology and came under the influence (in Physiology) of Leathes, one of the few people in my life whom I would unhesitatingly call a great man. Leathes also was a Fellow of the Royal Society before he ever came to Sheffield. His researches, especially on the physical chemistry of the fats, were recognized throughout the world. He was made a Fellow of the Royal College of Physicians in 1921 and gave the Croonian Lectures in 1923, and the Harveian Oration in 1930. Many distinguished research workers came to work with him and he was Dean of the Faculty from 1916 until 1922. He periodically invited the famous physiologists of the day to come and speak to us. In that way I met E. H. Starling, William Bayliss, J. S. Haldane (father of the more notorious J. B. S. Haldane), Joseph Barcroft and others who, although they may not have seen their own work in that light, were in fact forging the foundation of modern scientific medicine.

It must be confessed that it is difficult to recollect exactly what I learnt from them, but hearing great men speak with enthusiasm on their own subjects gives you inspiration. Bayliss,

I seem to remember, was the most relaxed and friendly, perhaps because he never had a medical qualification and the responsibilities which go with it. An amateur, one feels in retrospect, like some of the great founders of the Royal Society some two hundred and fifty years before him. Leathes and Starling, though perhaps more reserved, were friendly and not intimidating. Haldane was more difficult for the student to assess, and of Barcroft there are, of course, numerous anecdotes. Like Haldane, he was interested in the role of haemoglobin, and he became interested in the spleen at a time when little or nothing was known of its functions. It is said that he once asked a somewhat frightened candidate to tell him what were the functions of the spleen. After a few moments of panic the student blurted out, 'I'm afraid sir, I've forgotten.' 'Good Lord,' said Barcroft, 'now *nobody* knows.' Later, when he had become interested in the spleen's possible role as a regulator of the volume of circulating blood, he came to Sheffield to lecture on The Spleen to the Medico-Chirurgical Society. He started with the somewhat unexpected words, 'Ladies and Gentlemen, with the exception of the penis, the spleen alters its size more than any other organ of the body.'

But the whole of this period of my university education has to be seen against the grim background of the ghastly trench warfare of 1914–18. It went on and on and I suppose people of my age just accepted it as a way of life, and did not consider their future very seriously. I was envious of those a few years older than I who had faced the challenge of battle and, in fact, I volunteered in 1916 for military service, but my parents gave my true age and I was sent home on a charge of 'false attestation and misappropriation of the King's monies' (having accepted the customary King's Shilling on enrolment). When 1918 came and I was of proper age for military service I could have had an exemption on the grounds of being a medical student, but I preferred to take my part in active warfare with others of my generation. I had reached the rank of sergeant in the Officers' Training Corps at the University and now left the Medical School for training in No. 6 OCB (Officer Cadet Battalion) at Oxford and in six months qualified to be an Infantry Officer. I still hold the honorary rank of 2nd Lieutenant, I believe. I was due for service in France in the autumn of 1918, but the influenza epidemic was in full spate. I was struck down with it and my posting was postponed. A friend of mine in the same room also had the disease and one night I realized that he was very ill. He had the cyanosis (blue coloration) which became the sign of that type of influenzal pneumonia. I left my bed to send for the doctor, but my friend died the next day. That was, I suppose, my first experience of serious illness for I had not even reached the clinical stage of my medical training.

I was still on convalescent leave on November 11th, 1918, when the Armistice was signed. Influenza, which killed millions, may have saved my life, for the survival of an Infantry Officer in France at that time was precarious.

My other preoccupations throughout the medical course were Love and Music. Neither is specific to the Sheffield Medical School, but both are of great significance to my personal experience. Music will come into this narrative later. Of Love I must say that during my earlier years I was deeply in love with a girl called Lucie. Opportunities for intensive, passionate love-making were not what they are today. Landladies had a lower middle-class morality and a fear of getting a bad name by encouraging love-making amongst the unmarried. But Love will find a way. We danced together whenever we could; there was the back row of the cinema, and above all, because we were in Sheffield, there was the lovely quietude of the Derbyshire moors, the woods, the high bracken, and the mountain streams which darted underground and then reappeared. All this we explored and loved together. For a number of reasons it was not to endure.

And so because of Love and Music and War, my devotion to Anatomy and Physiology, despite the acknowledged quality of my teachers, was not as assiduous as it might have been.

Nevertheless I passed the necessary examinations, a few months late because of my brief military career, and I embarked on the clinical part of my course.

I remember standing at the bedside of a real patient for the first time. I even remember that he had pyloric stenosis and I am sure, though I might not have realized it at the time, that from then onwards I was a dedicated physician, and that this was a moment of intense importance and fulfilment in my life.

In most medical schools at that time students went straight from Anatomy and Physiology into a medical or surgical clerkship, in other words, an apprenticeship to a medical or surgical firm. Sheffield, innovatory as usual, was experimenting with an alternative in which the first six months (later I think reduced to three months) were spent in demonstrations and bedside teaching. I found this fascinating and from then on, despite my other preoccupations, found no difficulty in winning some high awards. We realized by speaking to students of some other medical schools that while they had twenty or thirty students round a bed, we had something much nearer to individual attention.

In the year following mine, Sheffield made another experiment, namely to start clinical work even before the examination in Anatomy and Physiology had been taken, so as to avoid the great dividing line between 'pre-clinical' and 'clinical' studies. I do not think this was very successful; students, however irrationally, like to feel that they have finished with something before embarking on something else, but the memory of this experiment was of great satisfaction to me about forty-five years later, when some of my colleagues on the Royal Commission on Medical Education were putting it forward as a new idea. The rest of our clinical course took the conventional form of a series of clerkships, in Medicine and Surgery, with three months in Gynaecology and Obstetrics and, during this time, we had lectures in Pharmacology and in Pathology.

When I was due to be a surgical clerk (actually called a dresser), the Royal Infirmary just after the War was so short of staff that I was actually invited to live in and act as House Surgeon to Mr Ernest Finch (later Sir Ernest) and supervise about fifty beds. Nevertheless, at the end of the time, despite inadequate leisure for study, I passed the third MB examination with distinction and a Gold Medal in Pathology. There is no doubt that my success was partly due to guile, because I realized that given enough self-assurance in a viva voce examination you could often lead the examiner away from an undesirable to a more desirable subject. I was delighted when I found this stratagem working with my External Examiner, who was Joseph Barcroft, himself a man of cunning.

Sheffield, like other non-collegiate universities of those days, had no halls of residence and so those students who could not live at home had to find lodgings. I was continuing my (still unfulfilled) endeavours to master the 'cello and the piano and always chose lodgings in which a reasonable piano was available. In those days when there was no radio and no very satisfactory gramophone, most middle-class homes had a piano.

What I have since called my policy of the calculated risk was put into full operation during my three months' clerkship in Gynaecology and Obstetrics. I witnessed, or assisted at twenty births, which was a requirement, but could not find much interest in the general subject of Gynaecology, which I had no intention of practising and which I thought could be adequately swotted up in six weeks before the final examination. During those three months I think I played the piano about four hours a day.

My landlady at that time was an attractive and passionate foreign woman who was ill-assorted with her rather vulgar husband, and much more attached to one of her lodgers. One day, when I was practising on her grand piano and cutting my lectures and attendances at the women's hospital, she came into the room to ask my advice. She wanted to discuss with me various ways in which she could murder her husband. I remember the occasion as a factual conversation without any obvious show of emotion. I rapidly realized that I might be deemed an accessory if I gave her any good advice and confined my attention to telling her the various ways in which her plans could be found out. I prize that memory as being My First Consultation. My Second Consultation was when her lover (back from the War) knocked her husband out and came to seek my opinion as to whether he was dead. Fortunately (for me at any rate) he was only concussed and already showing signs of recovery before I arrived on the scene. There must be few, if any, physicians whose first consultations were so challenging. Perhaps they were a good preparation for the life to come. At least I learnt the need for calm deliberation and self-control.

And now to return to my teachers. It must be remembered that there were three voluntary hospitals in Sheffield concerned with the teaching of the medical students: the Royal Infirmary, the Royal Hospital and the Jessop Hospital for Women. When I started clinical work as an undergraduate the chief Physicians were Hall (later Sir Arthur Hall) who was fifty-three, and A. E. Naish (forty-eight) at the Royal Hospital, and Barnes who, at the age of thirty-seven, was Senior Physician to the Royal Infirmary. We regarded Hall as rather a fatherly figure, whose teaching was less advanced than that of Barnes, but we always referred to him as Lord Arthur, a nickname of affection and respect. He was a dignified and significant figure in any society, but saved from being pompous by his irresistible sense of humour and subtle wit; and when I say irresistible I mean that he could not resist it himself, even though at times it might have been considered out of place. For instance, Sister Trevethick, who was the head of a nursing home at that time, told me how Hall was visiting one of his patients, a kindly old lady, who said to him, 'Dr Hall, if you and Sister can get me well again I shall be eternally in your debt.' 'I hope not,' said Hall, 'I don't like these eternal debts, I'd much rather that they paid spot cash.' The remark was not appreciated.

One of the many things, of great importance, which Hall did was to found what became the 'Arthur Hall Club', at which the honorary Physicians and Surgeons of all the teaching hospitals met to dine together from time to time, thus ruling out some of the old jealousies which had existed between the Royal Infirmary and the Royal Hospital. When Mellanby retired to become secretary of the Medical Research Council in 1934, the Club gave him a farewell dinner. Hall was in the chair. Sir Ronald Matthews, Chairman of the Governors of the Royal Infirmary was present as a guest. After the farewell speech in praise of Mellanby, Hall turned to Sir Ronald and asked him if he would like to say anything. Matthews rose and started by saying that he had not realized that he was going to be asked to speak, and then addressed us for what seemed like fifteen or twenty minutes, at the end of which Hall said, 'Sir Ronald said that he didn't know that he was going to be asked to speak' . . . pause . . . 'He certainly knew what he was going to say.'

There was one Professor whom Hall considered inadequate in his medical school, whom I will call Professor Ramsden. One evening Hall and Cobb (Ear and Throat Surgeon to the Royal Infirmary) were returning by taxi from the London train. As they passed the University Cobb remarked that the flag was flying at half-mast. 'Too much to hope that that's Ramsden I suppose,' said Hall.

Barnes was very modern in his outlook and had recently returned from Mesopotamia. He lectured in Pharmacology in addition to his teaching as a Physician in the wards. He taught us many things; for instance: that the most important disease in the world was malaria; that most of the drugs and complicated Latin prescriptions then still in vogue were useless; that some of them, such as Calomel, were positively poisonous; that there were only about seven (I think it was seven) medical remedies which had an established influence on disease. Those included (of course) quinine, also morphine and its derivations; thyroid extract; digitalis; mercury and salvarsan in syphilis;

iron (in certain anaemias) and with strict limitations atropine and bromide. There may have been one or two others, and later the new mercurial diuretics and quinidine were added.

I have already hinted that I discovered only later in life how out of date in comparison was the teaching in other medical schools. When, *some twenty-six years later*, I joined the staff of the Manchester Royal Infirmary as Professor of Medicine to the University, I remarked to one of the Senior Physicians, who also taught Therapeutics, that some of the students seemed to be lacking in knowledge of the basic principles of Medicine (meaning, of course, the application of Physiology to the understanding of disease). He replied, 'Yes I know, I asked one of them the dose of Calomel a few days ago, and he actually did not know it.' This is one of the occasions—I hope rare in my life—in which I lacked moral courage. Instead of saying, 'You're at least thirty years out of date', I changed the subject. It was, after all, important that as the University's first whole-time Professor of Medicine I should not start by making enemies.

Barnes soon became one of the moving spirits in the new outlook of the Sheffield Medical School and joined Hall and Leathes in the innovations which closely followed one another.

There was a vacancy on the staff of the Royal Infirmary owing to the retirement of its Senior Physician and in his place they appointed Edward Mellanby of all people who, though a thirty-six year-old medical scientist well-known for his experimental work on rickets, had no reputation as a clinician. This was revolutionary. He was given laboratories where he and his wife, May, could continue their experimental work. The University had the good sense to appoint as Mellanby's assistant, S. J. Cowell, who could supervise the clinical work of the unit. It was a bold experiment but certainly Mellanby brought to Sheffield the spirit of enquiry which was so lacking in most of the clinical schools of those days. Mellanby was really appointed Professor of Experimental Medicine, but because that title was unacceptable to the layman, he was called Professor of Pharmacology. Barnes gracefully retired from the lectureship which he had held in that subject and Mellanby took over the lectures. After all he had (according to the teaching of Barnes) only to learn up the actions of about seven drugs! And so the three full Physicians to the Sheffield Royal Infirmary were all under the age of forty. Finch, who was rapidly making his name as the leading Surgeon, was about the same age. I speak of 1920. (I qualified in 1921.)

There were other revolutionary appointments to come. When the Professor of Pathology, a skilled but conventional morbid anatomist, died, they appointed a young Australian experimental Pathologist to fill his place, namely Howard Florey.

My own clerkships, apart from the time when I was Student-House-Surgeon to Finch, were mostly spent at the Royal Hospital. There I learnt a great deal from that Scholar-Physician, Naish, who at the age of eighty-five left his home of retirement in Anglesey to come to London to cast his vote for me in the 1957 Presidential election of the Royal College of Physicians! I still proudly possess his open testimonial to me when I finished my term as his House Physician. Modesty (not one of my most notable attributes) forbids me to quote from it.

After qualification, I became House Physician to Hall and to Naish and then, after being a House Physician at the Royal Northern Hospital in London, I applied for the post of demonstrator in Pathology in Sheffield. After a year or two Barnes asked if I would become Medical Registrar to the Royal Infirmary, a post which they seemed to be creating for my benefit. Now I was under the tutelage of Barnes, Yates and Mellanby but, although Mellanby's influence on experimental medicine was supremely important to the Medical School, it was from Barnes that I learnt most. First because of his colossal knowledge of what was then the modern medicine and the new laboratory investigations which were becoming all-important in the diagnosis of disease, and second, because of his superb honesty and integrity. 'If you are concerned in new appointments,' he said 'always choose the best man. He may be a rival to you but in the long run we all benefit.' To my young mind this seemed to be unnecessary advice, but having since discovered in other medical schools the effects of nepotism coupled with a deliberate attempt to keep the best young men off the staff of the teaching hospital, I now know only too well what Barnes meant.

I must remind my readers that all staff appointments to teaching hospitals were then literally honorary, in the sense that there was no pay attached to them and you had to make your living through private practice.

Having served for some years as Medical Registrar to the Royal Infirmary, Barnes told me that they would make me Assistant honorary Physician as soon as I was ready—that is to say—as soon as I felt I could make a living. This they did in 1931, and when Mellanby left to become Secretary of the Medical Research Council in 1934 they made me full Physician, and appointed Wayne to succeed Mellanby on the experimental side with a more limited number of beds than had been allotted to Mellanby, which really were more than he needed.

When I was promoted to the honorary staff Barnes said to me, 'You'll see my mistakes and I'll see yours. Patients have a right to as many opinions as they like to pay for. Let us never fall out about it.'

Barnes was a great man, though not widely known outside Sheffield and its immediate environs. His interests were not limited to medicine. As someone said of another Physician who died recently, 'He was somewhat like Christ, J. He had great influence but never published anything.'

Thus around 1931 we had Leathes, Hall, Barnes, Mellanby and Florey all at the same time, which I think justifies my initial claim that the Sheffield Medical School was one of the most advanced in Britain, and justifies Hall's claim to my father that there was nothing I could learn in Edinburgh which they could not better teach in Sheffield.

I remember examining in Edinburgh some thirty years later and conducting a viva with one of their senior Physicians. It was his turn to question a rather shy Scottish lad. 'Tell me,' said the Physician, 'some of the signs of myxoedema' [hypothyroidism]. Long pause. No reply. Physician, encouragingly, 'Noo what about the weight? Would they no be gaining weight?' Long pause. 'Aye, they'd be gaining weight.' Pause. Physician: 'Well, would they no be feeling cold?' Long pause. 'Aye, they'd be feeling cold.' Pause. Physician: 'What about the hair? Would the hair no be dry and falling out?' Long pause. 'Aye, the hair would be dry and falling out.' Pause. Physician: 'Noo what about the pulse? Would the pulse no be slow?' Long pause. 'Aye, the pulse would be slow.' Time up. Exit student. Physician to me: 'He's a good chap that. I know his father very well—he's in general practice in . . .' (I forget where).

But to return to Sheffield, so great was the esteem of Leathes, Mellanby and Barnes that when insulin was first tried out in this country, and at first the licence to make it was closely guarded, Sheffield, and I think one other medical school, were the first to be allowed to do so. My wife, who qualified in medicine the year after I did, was then working in Leathes's laboratory and was given the job of actual preparation. The first patient was under the care of Barnes, his weight was about five stone. He had kept himself alive on a diet of cabbage and whisky. Thanks to insulin, he lived another thirty or forty years.

But for good measure, let me add that in Sheffield we had Naish and Yates, both extremely good and learned Physicians and teachers, and Rupert Hallam, a pioneer in the new approaches to Dermatology; and a genius in George Wilkinson, an ear and throat Surgeon, also a pioneer with neuro-surgical skills and a research worker on the mechanism of the cochlea of which he made his own models to show how it worked.

Also I was influenced as a student by R. G. Abercrombie. He was the head of the Edgar Allen Institute, devoted largely to the treatment of rheumatic complaints by physiotherapy. He was let loose on the final-year students from time to time.

He spoke impeccable English (his brother was Lascelles Abercrombie, Professor of English Literature in the University of Leeds). He introduced us to the psychological side of illness which in those days tended to be neglected. I am a fairly good Boswell and can often remember utterances with complete accuracy. I will give but two examples of his teaching, both concerned with the effect of deafness on illness. 'It is impossible to examine the abdomen of a deaf patient,' he said one day, thus making me realize how all-important is one's command of the patient during physical examination. And then, in relation to the difficulty of treating a deaf patient: 'The exhortations of the Physician, if uttered at the top of his voice, lose some of their power to persuade.'

Great as were many of my teachers, it was phrases such as these of Abercombie which had a lifelong effect in helping me to understand the patient, not merely his illness.

Other memories crowd in on me. Of course I went through experiences common to any medical student, which are yet unique to the individual. For instance, I hated Anatomy, particularly the dissection of the face of a corpse. I also dreaded my first operation and was worried that I might faint. For I had once fainted when I saw my mother open a blister with scissors. Yet when it came to that first operation, when I saw the Surgeon make a mighty incision into the abdomen of a fat woman with an umbilical hernia and the anaesthetized patient of course making no protest, it did not seem so horrifying. Yet to this day I avoid the operating theatre except when my presence there is of importance to my patient.

I suppose my fears were no greater or less than those of my contemporaries, though some fears medical students today would not have—such as those two contagious diseases: pulmonary tuberculosis and cerebro-spinal meningitis, both then essentially untreatable, though some patients, of course, recovered.

There were much more pleasurable experiences: not least the beautiful vision of young women unclothed to the waist—

visions given to artists and doctors in the course of their work. It is something which can be quite unrelated to desire or to sexual arousal—it is like viewing a Tiepolo Venus.

Finally, to return to my assertion of the greatness of the Sheffield Medical School. The staff of the Royal Infirmary lunched together, free of charge. There was no obligation to do so, but you would have been looked upon as rather a cad if you didn't lunch there with your colleagues about three times a week. Thus was harmony ensured between us. We could sort out our differences, if any, in a friendly way and, above all learn from one another. When I went to Manchester in 1946 I found that they had not yet reached that level of civilization. The consultants lunched at their clubs where the wealthy citizens were to be found. One surgeon might never meet another for weeks at a time. Manchester Medical School, of course, had its great men, three of them in fact. But if I were asked to catalogue without false modesty the important things I did in my twenty years at Manchester the initiation of a staff dining-room might well come first. Stupid indeed are administrators or bureaucrats who estimate these simple things in terms of cost-efficiency. The cost can readily be ascertained. The gains are untold.

Sir Derrick Dunlop

Sir Derrick Dunlop was born in Edinburgh in 1902, and educated at Oxford and Edinburgh. He was Professor of Therapeutics and Clinical Medicine and Physician to the Royal Infirmary, Edinburgh from 1936 to 1962, and is now Emeritus Professor. He was Physician to the Queen in Scotland, 1961–5, and is now Extra Physician. An Honorary Fellow of Brazenose College, Oxford, Sir Derrick has held numerous posts including that of Chairman of the British Pharmacopoeia Commission; Vice Chairman of the Regional Hospital Board, S.E. of Scotland; Member of the Scottish Secretary of State's Advisory Committee on Medical Research; Member of the Ministry of Health Committees on Food Policy and Drug Addiction; Chairman of the Ministry of Agriculture's Committee on Food Additives, etc. He has been editor of the Quarterly Journal of Medicine *and* Textbook of Medical Treatment, *and is the author of a number of medical papers and books.*

emory is of course a kindly thing: that of suffering tends to be evanescent while that of pleasure remains vivid; all the summers of long ago appear in recollection to have been most lovely and most temperate and even the winters of our discontent seem to have been days of bright sunshine glistening on ice and snow. Nevertheless, I know very well that I was extremely happy at my two medical schools of Oxford and Edinburgh. I was lucky to have been able to study medicine in two such beautiful cities.

How lovely it was going to Oxford in 1919 after the darkness of the First World War! It was not the traditional Oxford of Victorian and Edwardian times in which most of the undergraduates came straight from English public schools, but one drawing its student population from a rather wider spectrum of society. Besides ordinary freshmen like myself straight from school, many came up on their war gratuities, some of whom would not otherwise have come to Oxford at all. Ex-servicemen were allowed to qualify BA on a shortened course of two years. It was a very full Oxford with many older and more mature undergraduates, some of whom might have come up earlier had it not been for the interruption of the war. There were some who had been majors or even colonels and many who could strip their sleeves and show their scars.

At scarcely eighteen I must have been about the youngest

member of the University. My father had died in France during the war and I think my widowed mother was helped to send me to Oxford by one of his rich and grateful patients. I got £300 a year (there were plenty who had less) to cover everything including fees, food, accommodation, clothes, travelling and holidays. It is odd nowadays to recall that this kept me in modest comfort, though in the summer vacations I supplemented my allowance by hiring myself out for £3 a week and my keep as the tutor at some great house to teach little boys Greek and Latin. I did not enjoy very much being a sort of male Jane Eyre. It was an equivocal position as one never knew when to make oneself scarce or whether one was expected to pass the champagne at dinner.

At that time the Oxford medical school was a very small one. It only took some 30 to 40 undergraduates a year. It was then entirely a pre-clinical school and, after taking our BA degree in the Honours School of Natural Science—mostly in physiology —we had to do our clinical work elsewhere (the vast majority at the London teaching hospitals), going up to Oxford again for our later examinations. Of course there had been Regius Professors of Medicine at Oxford down the centuries and what a pageant they make! Sir Archibald Garrod, famed for his 'Inborn Errors of Metabolism' was Regius in my time. His predecessors included Linacre, Sydenham, Willis, Locke, Radcliffe, Acland and Osler. Nevertheless, till the school became a clinical one more recently, the Professor of Medicine was simply a senior administrative figure on the governing body of the University and was not involved in the active practice of medicine or in teaching undergraduates. In my day the Radcliffe Infirmary, now a medical centre attracting patients from all over the world, was little more than a glorified cottage hospital. The change is largely due to the Nuffield benefactions.

My fellow medical students included a considerable number of Rhodes scholars from what was then the British Empire, highly selected not only for their academic intelligence and character, but also for their sporting abilities. They were very fine fellows. Arthur Porritt, a Rhodes scholar from New Zealand, ultimately justified his selection by becoming a double blue, an Olympic runner, a well-known Surgeon in London, the President of the Royal College of Surgeons, Surgeon to Her Majesty, Governor General of New Zealand and a life peer. What a career! I confess I felt a bit out of my class among those people. There were also a few very able women students like Janet Vaughan who became a distinguished haematologist and Principal of Somerville College. In regard to female company, however, we then lived an almost completely monastic life during term time. Girls were then almost never seen in College except during Eights week or at the Commem balls. Only very occasionally when a mother or sister paid a state visit did our scouts go to great lengths in tidying our rooms and setting out a stately luncheon party in them with the College silver.

Brazenose was then a great sporting college full of blues and very hearty but not at that time a highly intellectual establishment. I look back on my four years there with undiluted delight and treasure my honorary Fellowship of it now with immense pride. The rugby football, the golf, the tennis, the punting on the Cher, the lovely surroundings, the splendid companionship and having one of those admirable old scouts to do one's bidding, were all enchanting. Nevertheless, the early study of medicine did not contribute greatly to this enchantment. Indeed I often wondered whether I had chosen the right profession. At school I had only studied the more humane letters and when I became a medical student I didn't know what H_2O was, far less C_2H_5OH. I must confess that elementary physics, inorganic chemistry and biology were most distasteful to me, especially as it was obvious that the often gifted scientists who instructed us found the teaching of the simplicities of their subjects to first-year medical students insufferably boring. I cannot recall that any of them attempted to instill into us the excitement of these approaches to science or of their relevance to our future practice of medicine. We would have welcomed that, just as we would have welcomed an occasional real doctor to talk to us on some of the clinical applications of these early studies. Further, I am sure we would have appreciated the physicist, inorganic chemist and biologist more had they again been introduced to us as occasional teachers in our more mature years. There is now an effort to break down the rigid departmentalism which then existed.

It sometimes seemed as though it was the function of the medical school to make us actively dislike the discipline to which we were exposed. The same sort of thing occurs to undergraduates in many other subjects. For example, students go to universities longing to plunge into the glories of English literature and, instead of starting them off on Shakespeare, Keats, Shelley, Jane Austen, George Eliot and Dickens, it is almost as though the authorities said to themselves, 'We'll soon take the smile off their faces' and put them to study for a year or so pre-Spenserian literature including the adventures of Piers Ploughman and Beowolf.

The next two years were occupied by anatomy, organic chemistry and physiology. I was not very fond of anatomy. Of course, those who are going to be surgeons must do individual dissections in preparation for the primary FRCS examination and learn detailed anatomy as postgraduates but it is doubtful whether all the anatomical minutiae we had to learn was necessary or whether the ordinary medical student at this stage should be required to dissect the whole body. I am certain I wasted a vast amount of time on my shocking dissections of it. I could learn so much more quickly and easily from good dissections done by experts, from models or from the exquisite blackboard drawings of the Professor of Anatomy—Arthur Thomson—with which he illuminated his rather dull lectures. He was a beautiful artist and his lectures on the human body at the Royal Academy in Piccadilly were I believe infinitely superior to those he gave us. One of his assistants was Alice

Chance—later as Mrs Carleton to become a well-known dermatologist. She was an admirable demonstrator but it is odd in this permissive age to remember my embarrassment at being taught about the human body by an attractive young woman. Nevertheless, the first really brilliant teacher I ever encountered as an undergraduate was Dr Whittaker at the Surgeon's Hall in Edinburgh to whom a few of us came from Oxford for a summer vacation course in anatomy. What a revelation he was! He taught anatomy by continually firing off questions to this or that member of his class. He usually treated our answers with mockery and ridicule. We never felt like going to sleep. I remember he once had me out kneeling before a female medical student to demonstrate the action of the patheticus muscle of the eye, as the levator palpebrae superioris was then sometimes called. Perhaps nowadays we are too frightened of a little histrionics in teaching, being apt to regard it as charlatanism and playing to the gallery. Students have to have some pegs on which to hang their memories.

Another drawback to the vast amount of time spent on dissecting and the minutiae of anatomy in my day was the tendency to start us learning everything by heart to the exclusion of making us think and appreciate general principles. Yet the pendulum of fashion, including that of education, always seems to swing too far at its extremes. The acquisition of many facts is inseparable from medical education, nor can one think about nothing in a factless vacuum. Modern educationalists seem to think it very wicked to teach little children to learn things off by heart. What nonsense that is! Provided they learn good stuff off by heart it does not matter much if they don't understand it very well at the time. 'Lead us not into Thames Station'—I used to imagine it as some dark sulphurous terminus! It is so easy to learn by heart in childhood and what one learns then remains fixed for ever even in the gathering mists of a senile memory.

After the awful hurdle of the first MB examination in anatomy and physiology had been surmounted we had to do an extra year taking a BA in Honours Physiology. It was a splendid course in which we ran round the Parks breathing into Douglas bags to the astonishment of the lieges and estimating afterwards our oxygen consumption and carbon dioxide production in Haldane gas apparatuses, inserting cannulae into the carotid arteries of anaesthetized cats and recording their blood pressures on smoked drums under a variety of influences, and so forth. During this year we fell under the influence of Professor Sir Charles Sherrington, one of the world's greatest physiologists and the worst and most incomprehensible of lecturers. Nevertheless, we felt it a privilege to work under such a great and good man and his brilliant colleagues—Haldane, Douglas, Priestley and Rudolph Peters.

I was so in love with Oxford that I wanted to stay there always. I thought there was just a chance that if I took a first in my Schools I might be elected to a Fellowship in my College and I worked hard though in my heart of hearts I knew I was no scientist. After the examination I remember travelling from London to see the results which were to be posted on a certain day. There were two nice American boys in my carriage in the train, rubber-necking round Europe, which was not so common then as it is now, and I said they must lunch with me in College and I would show them round Oxford. I put them into a hansom cab at the station (there were still a few such in Oxford then) which I thought would amuse them. Driving down the High I said as we got to the Schools, 'Do you mind if we stop here for a moment as there is something I want to see that I'm interested in?' I found that far from taking a first I had only just scraped through. I shall never forget the horror of that luncheon party trying to be cheerful and jolly with those two young Americans when I longed to get away by myself to nurse my misery.

Sometimes the apparent disasters in life turn out to be the great blessings. Instead of becoming a fifth-rate scientific don at Oxford I had to go back to Edinburgh to try to become a decent doctor. I must say, however, that when I returned home to do my clinical work I missed the weekly meeting with my erstwhile tutor—the famous or perhaps notorious J. B. S. Haldane. A few families like the Cecils, Churchills, Darwins and Huxleys go on breeding remarkable people for generations. Men of character and accomplishment have also emerged from the Haldane family. I found J.B.S.'s somewhat permissive views on sexual relations (they would seem very prosaic nowadays) extremely shocking—also his agnosticism and what seemed to me his very advanced liberal views on politics—just as he must have found the association with an immature, priggish, puritanical Scots youth extremely tedious. He did, however, explain what I had found bewildering in my lectures and criticized the weekly essay I had to write for him on a variety of subjects which made me a little more productive and less purely receptive. He also taught me how to use a library which at that time I would never have learned in Edinburgh. It was easy then in Oxford for each of the small numbers of medical students to have a personal tutor, but more difficult to arrange for this in medical schools with a far larger intake of students.

It was all very different when I returned to the great medical school of Edinburgh. Perhaps the torch of medical learning kindled by Hippocrates under his plane tree at Cos and which passed successively to Baghdad, Salerno, Montpellier, Padua and Leyden came to rest, for a while at any rate, in Edinburgh. There was a time in the first part of the nineteenth century when nearly a third of all the doctors practising in the then vast British Empire were trained in this comparatively small city.

There used to be a passion for learning in Scotland which in spite of its tiny population and grinding poverty supported four universities compared to England's two. Of the four Edinburgh is much the youngest. St Andrews, Glasgow and Aberdeen were pre-Reformation fifteenth-century foundations, whereas the University of Edinburgh was founded late in the seventeenth century—the Town's College as it was called. It was the first purely secular seat of learning in Britain. In England

Jews, Roman Catholics and non-Conformists were not then welcomed at Oxford or Cambridge which were also largely the preserves of the privileged classes. In consequence many emigrated to Scotland for their education and particularly to Edinburgh when it became the first university in Britain to provide a full training in medicine, just as centuries earlier students had flocked to Salerno, established by a Greek, a Roman, an Arab and a Jew. Although St Andrews and Aberdeen had for long granted medical degrees like Oxford, Cambridge and the Archbishop of Canterbury, no other British university at that time had a teaching medical school as Edinburgh had, whose Medical Faculty has recently celebrated its 250th anniversary. Not only was Edinburgh in the earlier part of the nineteenth century acknowledged to be the premier university medical school in the world but it had some claim to be the Modern Athens as well. Haydon the painter has described the scene: 'Princes Street with the castle radiantly illuminated by the setting sun; first you would see limping Sir Walter Scott with Lockhart his son-in-law; then the witty Dean Sydney Smith bear-leading his aristocratic pupils from London or Europe to the University; then trips Jeffrey of the *Edinburgh Review*, Adam the Architect and Raeburn the painter as if all had agreed to make their appearance at once.' It must have been so beautiful, too, for the elegant classic squares of the New Town still abutted on meadows, and the ancient pastures of Lord Moray's pleasure grounds north of Charlotte Square sloped down to thickets along the Water of Leith. You could look north to the Forth and Highland Hills over rustic meadows. The west wind still brought from the Pentland Hills the scent of moorburn in March and heather in August.

When I got back home to Edinburgh I received an invitation to a party given by the senior students of the University. It began, 'Dear Fresher, now that you are about to mount the Parnassus of learning. . . .' Young Oxford, with a newly acquired, if undistinguished, BA degree, found this very traumatic. Nevertheless, I soon settled down to a new clinical life. There were plenty of medical students who had homes, as I had, in the city, but the University of Edinburgh and its medical school have always had a cosmopolitan rather than a local population, drawing students from all over the world, particularly in those days when large parts of the British Empire had fewer universities and medical schools than they have now. Some students lived in three fine residential hostels —Ramsay Lodge, Blackie House and St Giles House looking to the north from the old town over Princes Street to the Forth and the hills of Fife. Most students, however, who came from outside Edinburgh lived in digs in the district of Marchmont, not far from the University, at an average cost of about £4 a week including breakfast and supper. The traditional Marchmont landladies were mostly kind, motherly figures and many students developed a warm friendship and attachment for them. For example, President Nyerere, when his country got its independence, had his old landlady out to Tanzania as his guest for the celebrations.

In 1923 the Edinburgh medical school was very large. The University took in 250 medical students a year and there were in addition a mass of candidates taking the triple qualification of the Royal College of Physicians, the Royal College of Surgeons of Edinburgh and the Faculty of Physicians and Surgeons of Glasgow. The clinical teaching of this concourse was all conducted in the wards of the Royal Infirmary except for infectious diseases, paediatrics and psychiatry. In popular clinics the crowd was so great that it was often necessary to stand on a bench to catch a glimpse of the patient under discussion. No wonder that every hour of our day had to be organized from morning to night, but as far as I can remember, we were perfectly happy to be so regimented.

Besides practical laboratory classes and clinics in the wards there were three or four lectures to attend every day at which it was the object of the Professor of each subject to teach in his course of lectures the whole of pathology, pharmacology, bacteriology, therapeutics, medicine, surgery, obstetrics and gynaecology, psychiatry, paediatrics, public health and forensic medicine. In addition there were comprehensive courses of lectures on the special subjects of dermatology, venereal diseases, tuberculosis, oto-rhino laryngology, and ophthalmology. The lectures were mostly very competent but we certainly had a surfeit of them. If one was regular in attendance and a good note-taker there was no need to read much to pass the examinations as long as one could decipher the notes and commit them sufficiently to memory. There we would sit for long hours each day, poised over our note books, and when the lecturer came in and said 'Good morning' we got that down too. This sort of thing persisted till after the last war! I well remember when I became a Professor in 1936 how often some pathetic little joke I may have made in a lecture reappeared afterwards in examination scripts. One felt on reading them a little like a dog returning to its own vomit.

There are changing fashions in teaching as in clothes, and lectures are now utterly decried by the moderns. Of course, we then had far too many lectures, but it is possible to denigrate them excessively in favour of small group teaching. There are many broad principles that can be imparted just as well to scores of students in a lecture theatre as to five in a tutorial and with a great saving of teaching time. Further the spoken word of a good lecturer—with possibly a tinge of histrionics— can often be made more memorable than the written word. Lectures should excite, stimulate and amuse, leaving in the mind of their audiences only two or three important principles with a wealth of illustrative examples, and indicate the literature on the subject which should be read. They should not attempt to be comprehensive or to take the place of textbooks, as they tended to be at that time in Edinburgh, or to cram the mind with facts like those excessively elaborate lantern slides whose complicated graphs and tables may be quite clear to the speaker who has pondered over them for ages but quite incomprehensible to his audience when flicked on and off every few moments.

In my time as a student and young doctor, Edinburgh was one of the world's great surgical schools. Inspired originally by Sir Harold Stiles, Sir John Fraser, Sir David Wilkie and Sir Henry Wade became surgeons of international repute with very able colleagues and assistants. I confess that the amount of time we students used to spend watching these great men operating from the galleries of warm, rather sleep-making theatres was often a little wasted. As I could never tie a knot and was quite handless I was not tempted to become a surgeon but was very much attracted to clinical medicine. Perhaps the Edinburgh physicians were not then as distinguished as their surgical colleagues but there were some interesting characters among them, particularly my future chief, Sir Robert Philip; not perhaps a great clinician so much as a great medical statesman especially in the field of tuberculosis. He could have been an equally distinguished prince of the church, foreign secretary or a tycoon of industry.

Good history-taking constitutes fully 70 per cent of clinical medicine and most of its art. It involves the art of communication between doctor and patient and forms the quality which makes one say 'that man is a good doctor'. After an accurate history has been elicited, the diagnosis and subsequent management of the patient, too, usually become fairly obvious. The ability to take a good history can only be taught properly by example to small groups of students sitting not standing round a bed. It is true that there have been a few geniuses who can render the patient they are interviewing entirely oblivious to a large audience in a lecture theatre so that they will talk of their most intimate affairs as though they were alone with their interlocutor. Sir David Henderson who became the distinguished Professor of Psychiatry in Edinburgh shortly after I qualified had to a remarkable degree this very rare, almost hypnotic ability.

We were taught history-taking pretty well in Edinburgh but, as in most other schools at that time, its value was overshadowed somewhat by the determining influence of the final clinical examination. At it the main emphasis used always to be centred—and still may be for all I know—on the recognition of physical signs such as gross cardiac murmurs, pupils that had long since failed to react to light, spleens spreading into the right iliac fossa and pulmonary cavities sighing out their amphoric breath sounds to the accompaniment of consonating crepitations and whispering pectoriloquy—'good teaching cases' as they were called—and lists of those exhibiting such desirable features were kept, and the patients were whistled up for the finals, but they were cases that the student would seldom see again. Thus on going into practice subsequently we were apt to feel like the evil and adulterous generation seeking a sign and no sign was vouchsafed unto us. There are always plenty of physical signs to be found in any patient but not often those patent ones, on the elicitation of which so much time and effort was then expended in the wards.

The trouble is that if a large number of students has to be assessed in a limited time at the final examination it is easy to make up one's mind in a few minutes on a candidate by his ability, or lack of it, to appreciate a loud aortic diastolic murmur and a water hammer pulse; but one would be more hesitant in coming to a conclusion if he failed to appreciate the significance of a middle-aged man complaining of some loss of memory and early morning nausea, with not very much in the way of physical signs save a slightly tremulous hand and a single small spider web naevus on his nose which could be so easily missed.

Though I had plenty of theory drummed into me I found it difficult in the Royal Infirmary to get sufficient practical clinical experience in personally handling patients because of the large number of students which then crowded the wards. Consequently I answered an advertisement for a student clinical assistant in the large poor-house parish hospital in Edinburgh. I was successful in obtaining the appointment. In exchange for my keep I had to assist in minor duties in the wards before leaving for work in the morning and again on returning from my classes in the evening. The place then still retained many of the attributes of the workhouse in which Oliver Twist was born. Two resident women doctors were responsible for all the patients in the hospital's acres of rather forbidding wards, smelling slightly of excrement mingled with the odour of iodoform, carbolic and oil of sassefrass which was used to dress the almost invariably verminous heads of the patients on admission. My two mistresses with whom I lived (I hasten to add that they were middle-aged and by no means delicately wanton) worked me hard but I had a marvellous clinical experience. I soon found out, however, that my real raison d'être was to pass catheters on a number of old men early each morning, and also when I got back in the evening when the poor things were nigh bursting, for it was not considered decent that my mistresses should condescend to this essential if embarrassing duty. One of them would always say before breakfast and supper, 'Will you ask a blessing please, Mr Dunlop', upon which I would intone, 'Oh Lord, for these the least of thy mercies make us suitably thankful.' The poor-house meals were the least of his mercies, though since then I have regarded the pleasures of the table as among his greatest blessings.

No memories of the Edinburgh medical school would be complete without a reference to the Royal Medical Society. Founded in 1732 by a few young men chattering in a tavern it has since been a centre for debates by medical students, for the reading of papers by them and for communications to the Society by distinguished visitors. It is the oldest medical society in Britain, certainly the only undergraduate one with a royal charter, and has contributed enormously to the social and intellectual life in Edinburgh of its members. Besides contributing considerably to our medical education the Society did much to make us less inarticulate, to speak and to conduct public business. I remember it with great affection.

What an undertaking the final examinations were! Nearly three weeks of a concentrated hell of papers and clinicals covering a wide variety of subjects. Perhaps as the result of my poor-house experience I did reasonably well and was gloriously capped in the MacEwan Hall in full evening dress in the presence of admiring friends and relations. I got a £100 prize which made life much easier, and as two months had to elapse before my first house appointment I hired myself as house physician to a ducal house party in the North of Scotland where in addition to my splendid keep I got £7 a week—over twice my salary as a tutor—and had nothing to do but fish and shoot. It was great to be a real doctor at last.

William Sargant

Born in London in 1907, William Sargant was educated at Leys School and St John's College, Cambridge, before going to St Mary's Medical School in 1928. He has held various posts, including House Surgeon to the Surgical Professorial Unit, House Physician to the Medical Unit, Medical Superintendent and Assistant to the Medical Unit, St Mary's Hospital; Physician, Maudsley Hospital; Rockefeller Research Fellow, Harvard Medical School; Physician in Charge of the Department of Psychological Medicine, St Thomas's Hospital; Registrar, Royal Medico-Psychological Association; Associate Secretary, World Psychiatric Association. He is the author of Battle for the Mind *(1957), and is now Honorary Consulting Psychiatrist, St Thomas's Hospital.*

I have had the good fortune to be connected with four widely different Medical Schools. Coming down from Cambridge in 1928, I completed my medical qualification and later obtained my MRCP at St Mary's Hospital, London. If I concentrate on this part of my career it is not only because it is so fascinating to me, but because it should interest others, for St Mary's official history is formal and by no means gives one complete glimpses of the medical students' life at that time.

My first contact with St Mary's had already begun at Cambridge. A Dr Charles Wilson (later to become the famous Lord Moran) visited us in his little snub-nosed Austin car. He explained to me that, as Dean, he was trying to build up St Mary's Medical School by offering scholarships to all-rounders —those who were good at games and who were also reasonably intelligent. I came into this category: I had played several times for the University at rugby and was Captain of the College Team; I had become President of the Cambridge University Medical Society; and I was on the Committee of the Cambridge Union along with Lord Caradon, Gilbert Harding, the late Lord Crowther and others who later would do well in life (I first spoke at the Cambridge Union when Lord Devlin was its President).

So I had the qualifications Dr Wilson was looking for. He wanted *people who kept going*. How right he was can be seen in retrospect, for so many of his 'Games Scholars', including Lord Porritt, got on to the staff, later, of the London teaching hospital's. Not that being good at games was his sole criterion for bringing students to St Mary's. He had the good sense to choose people like Professor Henry Barcroft (recently retired from St Thomas's) who had outstanding academic personalities, though no proven skill at games.

St Mary's was in a terrible way when I arrived. Few students had come there from Oxford or Cambridge, they preferring, more sensibly, Guy's or Bart's or The London. Indeed, such was the poor reputation of St Mary's that the University Grant's Committee had threatened it with closure as a teaching hospital. It was this that prompted Charles Wilson to institute a Medical and Surgical Professorial Unit, so that apart from part-time Harley Street consultants there would always be staff available for teaching purposes. By forming such a Unit, Charles Wilson was a pioneer. Yet this move was not entirely a disinterested one, for Wilson became the first Assistant to the Medical Unit as well as Dean—and he drew a salary, though rarely, in fact, did he teach. When he did so, he was absolutely brilliant at it.

St Mary's had not only been badly organized from the point of view of teaching, but the buildings, too, were decrepit. The Medical School was simply a house near the Paddington Canal, and the students' dirty recreation rooms were in the hospital cellars and disgracefully furnished. No wonder there were few students and many of these were young Welsh boys 'let loose', away from home for the first time and living in sordid Paddington. Opposite Paddington Station was a row of shabby hotels in whose registers the forged names of senior members of St Mary's staff appeared with consistent regularity! Praed Street itself, where St Mary's stood, was also in a low condition with its birth-control shops and public houses of dubious reputation.

In 1928, when I arrived, St Mary's even had an appalling rugby fixture list. This meant much travelling to South West

England until we later on got good London fixtures. I never felt really at home with my rugby colleagues who rejoiced in alcohol and in the ritual debagging of frightened team members on the way back in the train. I made my way to a Barbarian cap more by the use of my wits as a forward than brawn. (I gave up football soon after qualifying, not wishing to become labelled as a 'rugger tough'—I wanted to get down to serious medicine and research.)

Yet, considering everything, ten years after the First World War had ended, the morale of the School was good. There were some extraordinary students there. Some were shell-shocked survivors of the War; some were taking Medicine for special purposes—to join an exploratory expedition, for example; some were receiving incomes from bequests and did their best to keep the money flowing by not qualifying. One student failed his finals ten times; yet later he became a careful and respected Oxford practitioner.

Apart from Wilson's scholars all had to pay tuition fees and because no one was paid for the great honour of getting a job at one's own teaching hospital, I can only remember one person getting married while a houseman. Incidentally, Dr Wilson stopped women being admitted to St Mary's as so many got married after qualifying—it seemed part of his plan to build up the hospital's reputation by their exclusion!

Eventually, I became very friendly with Wilson. I had become Captain of St Mary's football and had played for the champion county Middlesex, and for London and, as I've said, for the Barbarians. He came to most of the games and invited me often to his house. Though many hated him at St Mary's and at other medical schools, I had a great admiration for him. He would return to Harley Street having been outvoted at Committee meetings, very depressed, and saying he was going to resign as Dean. His intelligent and most charming wife would say, 'Don't—that's just what they want you to do.'

He repeatedly said he could not build up St Mary's simply by giving academic scholarships. He was very anxious we should win the Rugby Cup. He knew that if we did so students would choose St Mary's, as they knew little enough generally about London hospitals. They would assume that if St Mary's kept winning the Cup it must be a good medical school. He was right. And he was also right in linking Paddington Infirmary with St Mary's in order to provide first-class teaching material and jobs for students.

An important ally in Charles Wilson's endeavours to make St Mary's a successful and prestigious School was Lord Beaverbrook. I was in the Dean's house in Harley Street when he returned to say he had just been called in by Beaverbrook to examine the young Max Aitken. When he had disagreed with the other doctors at the consultation he had been curtly dismissed. 'But I'll be called back in a month,' he said. And he was. Afterwards, he continued to look after Beaverbrook himself as well as Lord Castlerosse who introduced him to Churchill. Thus the future great war partnership of Churchill and Lord Moran began.

Wilson persuaded Lord Beaverbrook to give a large sum of money for a new medical school and for a very large library. 'The bigger the library, the more students will come,' he insisted. And again he was right.

Apart from Charles Wilson, the clinical staff was not of high standard. And many of them were at war with each other— unless they closed ranks to attack the Dean. Colleagues from the other hospitals were calling them rugger professionals when they met, and they resented it. Among the staff at that time was Sir William Wilcox—a self-made doctor with an enormous practice success. He believed most illnesses derived from focal sepsis so, as a result, hundreds of normal teeth were needlessly extracted from suffering patients. One of the jobs of Sir William Wilcox's assistants was to try and explain to patients why their good teeth had to come out when Sir William's filthy teeth stayed in! Focal sepsis has now gone out of fashion, and it is wonderful what doctors will believe in with so little proof. But it made large fortunes for several members of the staff and staff members were even elected because of their work in it and stayed on working at it for years after it was discredited.

The then unknown Alexander Fleming also must have been making a fortune at that time preparing individual vaccines for patients, but using these vaccines afterwards in his laboratory. I voluntarily worked in this laboratory and watched Fleming dabbing wounds with penicillin until he gave up this practice. Sir Almroth Wright would not let Fleming inject the penicillin because he believed that if the germs were killed off, then the body's defence mechanisms would be adversely affected. Ten years were wasted before Chain and Florey injected penicillin at Oxford. Then, Fleming, who had really wanted to be a surgeon and was a disappointed man, became an everlastingly famous world figure.

Coming under some old regulations I qualified MRCS, LRCP in two years and took an MB one year later. It was not a happy time for me. My father, who had been very rich in the City, in the 1928–29 slump was facing bankruptcy, which he just avoided. Financially I just scraped through my medical student days because of my games scholarship, even though I wasn't well, having then an undiagnosed attack of severe tuberculosis. But one had to keep going, as Wilson said.

On qualifying, I worked at first as House Surgeon to the Surgical Professorial Unit under Dixon Wright and Lord Porritt. The former was to some extent a genius and a tremendous character, always trying out new methods and new ideas. He saved so many lives and did so much for British and international surgery, yet when he died recently, though world famous, not one single honour of any sort had been bestowed upon him. I learned, early, that one did not get on in medicine by being a good doctor, but for political and social reasons. Even Fleming's knighthood was given late, and reluctantly. Florey, the administrator, on the other hand, was given a peerage. But helping patients brings the greatest happiness in life, not playing at medical power politics, not sitting on forty or more committees in order to receive honours and awards.

I sayed on at St Mary's doing general medicine till 1934, when somebody else got the staff job I should have liked. I had to choose either a speciality or go into general practice. Though I never intended initially to go into psychiatry, I think I have done more good eventually in this speciality than I would ever have done by staying in general medicine. While at St Mary's I had read for my membership of the Royal College—so essential if one wished to reach consultant status, but so difficult then to obtain. When I passed this examination at my first attempt Wilson was delighted.

By the time I left St Mary's, much of what Wilson had hoped for had come to pass. An ever-increasing quota of students from Oxford and Cambridge were coming to the School, and it was soon to have a high academic record as well as a sporting one. So the future Lord Moran was right about games scholarships—and he was right, too, about Games Scholars. They kept on fighting to the end, not only for themselves, but also for their patients.

Ellia Berstock

Ellia Berstock was born in Dublin in 1915 and when only 14 entered the medical school of the Royal College of Physicians and Surgeons, Dublin. After a brilliant student career he qualified in 1937. Subsequently he worked in Longton Cottage Hospital and then for a short spell in Stockport Infirmary before entering general practice taking assistantships in Nottinghamshire, Sheffield and the Doncaster–Maltby area. In 1945 he became single-handed general practitioner of a large practice in Stockport, where he has remained ever since. During his leisure time he is a collector of antiques (particularly of Netsuke), and he still plays cricket. He is currently engaged on his autobiography, and from the first draft of this work-in-progress the following chapter has been extracted.

The young doctor walked down Arnott Street towards The Meath Hospital. Through the curtained window of our parlour we saw him stop on the edge of the pavement, and with a solemn obsequious flourish, raise his hat to the herd of cows that was being shepherded through the street. The young farmhand in charge smote the streaming backsides of the animals with his short stick and adroitly avoided the dung which the creatures were profusely shedding. All our neighbours—my father too—avidly gathered with buckets and shovels the manure that would soon help along the rhubarb and make the nasturtiums thrive. In spite of all this activity I knew, though I was only a small boy, that my mother had only eyes for the young bowing doctor. For above all, my mother admired those who belonged to the medical profession. Was she not always talking about the doctors of her era—Sir John Moore, Drs Boxwell, Crofton and Muirhead, Drs Barrie and Bethel Solomons? 'A doctor is so well respected,' she always said.

My mother had always been close to illness. She had been ill herself and early in her marriage she went through the trauma of nursing my fair-haired, blue-eyed brother who was to die at the age of one year. So if I am a doctor today, it is mainly because of all these early years of conditioning. Of course I think I also wanted to help in the ever-dwindling fortunes of my family and perhaps I hoped, too, that somehow by becoming a doctor I could halt the deterioration of my mother's health. Yet, if I was asked in 1930 what I wanted to be, I would have replied without hesitation, 'A writer.' My mother listened to my 'blank verse' and she would approve and encourage me even more openly to write than she would about medicine; but there was a tacit agreement between us that there was no future in being a poet or a writer. It wasn't solid enough. The pit-falls, my mother indicated, were tremendous. One had to get a degree and no degrees were issued to poets. So I began to look upon my desire to write as a luxury, a refuge, something secondary to the task of becoming a doctor.

And so it came about that I was one of the youngest, if not the youngest student to obtain entrance to the medical school of the Royal College of Ireland. There I was, a lean lad of fifteen, cutting up and dissecting dead bodies. I remember feeling quite hopeless and morbid as I picked at the nerve roots and the white tendons of some unfortunate vagrant. Entering medical school is not the same as entering other departments of a university. The subjects are all completely charted, all plotted. No vibrant discussion can take place about the vagus nerve or its origin, its branches, or what muscles it enervates. One cannot have an opinion about it as, say, a student studying English Literature may have about a poem by Shelley. The functions of the stomach or the thymus gland were already formulated. We just had to learn and remember. Indeed there were few *why's* and *wherefore's* about any subject throughout the whole medical student curriculum—and this to my mind is one of the main causes of the medical profession's mediocrity. All one needs to be successful as a medical student is a good memory and an aptitude to pick out the essentials and a capacity to build around them in order to pass examinations.

I applied myself with great determination and I had some good teachers: Professor Evelyn J. Evatt and Billy Whelan and 'Garry' who would weigh a skull in the palm of his hand and dryly remark, 'Alas, poor Yorick.' And I admired Professor Jessop who would enter our tiered lecture room, gown flowing, ruddy-faced, resembling Joshua Reynolds's portrait of Oliver Goldsmith. I am proud to have been one of his pupils. Yet in spite of all my industry, my compulsion to study, my interests were many and interwoven with the city of my birth—Dublin. I was not like other students, jerked out of an earlier environment to take digs in an unknown city with an unknown people. I lived at home in Arnott Street with my family until I passed the Anatomy and Physiology examinations. Soon after, it is true, my family moved to Sheffield and I stayed in my grandparents' home in Victoria Street. From then onwards my student career was punctuated by telegrams (now yellowed) of congratulations from my mother and father and family in England. I must say that I regret my mother never *directly* shared my successes of which she was the architect.

I am speaking of the 'thirties when the new State was finding its strength, when De Valera and Cosgrave strode the scene, when tariffs and embargoes were enforced not only on agricultural and industrial products, but there were even whispers of restrictions in allowing doctors to emigrate and practise in England. This was particularly worrying to the medical student population of Dublin as there were not enough posts to soak up the immense turn-out from the three medical schools. They did not realize that England could manage without Irish pigs but not without Irish doctors.

Meanwhile because of my slogging I passed the cruel marathon Anatomy and Physiology examination. I did well and was appointed student demonstrator in both subjects and also in Histology (and was awarded first prize and medal).

I had now reached the stage where I was expected to pick the hospital in which I desired to do my internship. There was a great choice because hospitals, like churches, pepper the city of Dublin. I chose the Royal City of Dublin Hospital—known to students as Baggott Street Hospital. I recall my first visit to the surgical ward. I was amazed and distressed to see the patients entwined in weird contraptions, so that they would be hung and strung up with traction applied to their lower limbs —all suspended in mid-air by pulleys and wires. I was to see this Hogarthian scene repeated in the wards of all the hospitals I attended. For these were the bad years before milk had to be compulsorily sterilized and when bone tuberculosis was the arch-enemy of the rural population.

I often visited The Meath Hospital to listen to Dr Murphy, a perky man, fly-collared and pin-stripe suited. One morning he demonstrated a case of hysterical paralysis. Dr Murphy made this patient walk—albeit temporarily—by applying a red-hot metal disc to the patient's backside. To our amazement the paralyzed patient jumped out of bed to walk speedily around the ward like an automaton or as in a silent film of Charlie Chaplin. To heighten our surprise the patient did not complain of the pain of being branded.

Witnessing such scenes made me feel that I had wandered into a new world where in different hospitals I could see for myself the misery of human beings and appraise the stoical attitudes which they revealed despite tremendous hazards and impending defeats. At this time I was clerk to Dr Alfred (Alfie) Parsons, a bluff, eccentric, elderly gentleman who always expected me to deliver a diagnosis by inspection alone—the furrows of a patient's forehead indicated a peptic ulcer, or a stick beside the bed suggested hemiplegia. My time was so fully occupied in working for Alfie Parsons that now I cannot recollect the other consultants apart from Mr Stoney for whom I did a surgical clerkship and Mr Pringle (I nicknamed him Perineal Pringle because he performed heroic and gargantuan operations it seemed always through the perineum) and two or three others, including Dr Synge who was related to J. M. Synge and like him had a high forehead, drooping moustaches and a sallow de-energized face.

It was not all work. There was the Baggott Street Hospital

annual dinner, held in the Gresham Hotel, when I drank the Pol Roger 1929 as if it were water. That night 'Jammie' Clinch, the famous gentle giant of Irish rugby football, who was also in residence—had to put me to bed. And the Christmas dinner, I fear, shamefully and deplorably, ended in a battle of food between the residents and the junior staff. Custards, blancmanges, fruits, nuts, potatoes were fired at each other, and the matron vowed never again to supply the residents with such good fare. Our protest against surfeit was duly acknowledged.

One evening, whilst I was on Casualty duty, three men unsteadily presented themselves. One of these was the sports editor of the *Irish Independent* who had written about my cricket performance in glowing terms in the Sunday edition. He had caught his finger in the door of his motor car and it was necessary to clean the wound and insert stitches. The second man, a small bowler-hatted rotund figure turned out to be no other than 'Buck Mulligan'—Dr Oliver St John Gogarty—he was half sober. The third man, they called Dr Murphy. After my bit of surgery, I was pressed to join them for further refreshments. I well remember Oliver St John Gogarty's critical asides as, with cruel dispassion, he plied his two drunken friends with more and more tots.

We were expected to attend a number of lectures about mental illness and so with reluctance I visited the Grange Gorman Mental Asylum, which like some unclean thing was situated outside Dublin City. There I saw, for the first time, the tortuous twists the mind can take. I saw poor souls condemned in a vast prison, committed without the semblance of a chance of ever returning to their homes. Grange Gorman will always live in my memory as a sad place, entombed, where the inmates pathetically took imaginary round-the-world trips, carrying their possessions in battered cardboard suitcases strapped around with trailing string. Then there were those, not journeying, but solemnly pronouncing doom and those who believed that their mission was to repeat the Sermon on the Mount. Yet others had suffered a metamorphosis and had been, as it were, transfigured into animals both real and imaginary—all these poor patients hidden away outside the city walls, outside the pale, something buried, unwholesome, saddening and forlorn.

Having finished my residency in Baggott Street Hospital, there were the Cinderella subjects of Medical Jurisprudence and Toxicology, Materia Medica and Ophthalmology to pass, and indeed I was to win first prize and medal in some of these examinations. Next in our curriculum was Pathology and Bacteriology. Our Professor was Boxwell, a patriarchal figure, grey-haired and grey-moustached. His book *Boxwell and Purser* was not standard reading but it was breathless and breezy and a much less stereotyped textbook than those currently used. He was a most original lecturer, and his asides were gems to be treasured. He was so enthusiastic about the role that Pathology played in the correct practice of Medicine and Surgery that his face glowed with uninhibited reverence when he peered into the glass jars containing, in formaldehyde, a heart, or a kidney, a liver or a lung. I again was successful in passing the Pathology examination and was awarded first prize and medal.

It was time now to decide at which Maternity Hospital I was to do my residence. My friend, Hymie Sharpe, and I went through all the details and decided against the Coombe Maternity Hospital, for it lacked lustre, and we rejected Hollis Street also, because it was a comparatively new unit. We chose the Rotunda (what an apt name) which had a world-wide reputation and which drew students from all the continents, as well as many doctors intent on doing postgraduate work. Dr Davidson, the Master, was a quiet, phlegmatic, impersonal and methodical clinician; he had sway over this vast complex. His word was law—his being sacred. He *was* the custodian of the Rotunda's fame. Hymie Sharpe and I pooled our meagre financial resources and managed to purchase the necessary equipment—a Gladstone bag, of which we were truly proud, a good supply of tow (substitute for cotton wool), umbilical string, a female catheter, a mucous extractor, and gloves. Ergot would be supplied by the hall porter or by the district midwife.

Students were required to attend twenty deliveries outside the Hospital—'on the district'—and witness, in the hospital, a number of gynaecological and obstetrical operations. On the district we were to be assisted by the district midwife and we could call out the clinical assistant from the hospital if we felt there was any danger to child or mother. We were placed on a rota. So when our names were near the top of the list we had to be in or near the hospital waiting. Hymie and I decided to take up residency during the last three months of the year when, with luck, the twenty deliveries would be done within a matter of weeks.

The Rotunda Hospital was situated at the end of O'Connell Street on the way out of the city towards Phoenix Park. It was surrounded by tenement houses which had once, in the eighteenth century, been the houses of the privileged classes. Now seedy and run-down, they still bore the unmistakable traces of neo-classical architecture with pillared entrances above which archways enclosed expansive fanlights, and panelled front doors from which the brass furnishings had long ago disappeared. The wide stairways and sweeping banisters still gave some hints of past glory and elegance. With my friend Hymie, I would sit in Mooney's bar which was conveniently situated across the road from the Rotunda. It was always half filled with the local population and half with students from America, Canada, South Africa, India, New Zealand and Australia who had come to enlarge their knowledge of Obstetrics and Gynaecology, but who also became conversant with Guinness and John Jameson and that particular brand of ritual that belongs solely to the Rotunda.

Soon our names appeared on the rota and I checked our purchases. The Gladstone bag was missing! Hymie, who liked a flutter on the horses, could not account for its disappearance. I had a feeling that its deep black glossy leather was reposing on the top shelf of a pawnbroker's shop. The bag had gone irrevocably, the bag that was to have been the emblem of our status.

So without it we hurriedly packed the instruments and tow into brown paper and set off on our first mission towards Gardiner's Street. It was raining. We arrived at the tenement bedraggled, our brown paper parcel a wet, unfriendly mess. No matter, the patient was well and all was going well. This was going to be her fifth child. Then, suddenly, not long before the baby's head was crowned, all the lights went out. The mother shrieked, the nurse shouted, and a multiple cry went out for money for the gas meter. We two would-be doctors fumbled in our pockets uselessly. Nobody seemed to have any money. The poor husband was violently berated. Candles, a commodity stocked in every Irish home, were brought into the room, lighting the mother on the bed. In this subdued light the squawking baby was immediately born, to the delight of all the family and all the neighbours. We were feted and praised and given large cups full of the hard stuff. 'Gawd have mercy upon you, doctor.' 'Have a drink wid me.' 'Gawd bless you, doctor', and the old grandmother too would join in with 'May the Laurd give you and yours good health and may the Blessed Virgin look down upon you.' The father's voice followed us down the stairs, 'Gawd bless you doctor', and we were proud that we had successfully kept the Rotunda's fame and name from being disgraced. The poor of Dublin made us feel as if we were champions. And my admiration for the women of Ireland with their brood of children, and their great concern for family life, remains to this day undiminished.

I enjoyed my residency at the Rotunda though the bell would toll at any hour of the night or day—in bedroom, in dining-room, even in the toilet, to summon us to the operating theatre to witness the Master, Professor Davidson, or Assistant

Master perform an intricate obstetrical procedure or a caesarian section. Tired, clothes hastily pulled over our pyjamas, some in slippers, we would wend our way to the gallery of the theatre to peer down at Dr Davidson or young Edward Solomons (nephew of Bethel Solomons) swathed in white and green extracting another little caesar from the warmth of his mother's womb.

But my days at the Rotunda, indeed all my student days, were enacted against the backdrop of Dublin. The Rotunda itself was ideally situated near the city, and not far from the North Wall, from Joyce's Nighttown and Lord Longford's Gate Theatre. I recollect Lord Longford's large Pickwickian form emerging from the Gate, and at other times we would catch glimpses of Hilton Edwards and Michael MacLiammoir. I was conscious too, of the proximity of Liberty Hall, The Engineers' and Apprentices' Hall, geographical landmarks of the uprising, and I was proud to be in the environs of places of such historical moment. As a student, I was wrapt in the nostalgia of the recent past and had a great sympathy with those who, in these very places, made their contribution to the remaking of the city of Dublin.

My friend, David Robinson, who had just qualified as a dentist would call for me and we would make our way to the Abbey Theatre. On one occasion we walked together in a torchlight procession to listen to De Valera speak outside the GPO. I made many trips at night into the heart of the City whilst I was resident in the Rotunda—if not with Davy Robinson, then with Hymie Sharpe and a couple of South African students. We eyed the girls and more often than not casual acquaintanceships developed and we would walk to secret places in Phoenix Park.

Having completed twenty deliveries in just under a month, I was sorry to have to return to my grandparents' home. I enjoyed every minute of my short stay at the Rotunda: it broadened my outlook and made me realize how international the art of medicine was. At the same time it was comforting to know that one was being equipped with a skill and knowledge that in future years would help one to help others. I again passed the examination and was awarded first prize and medal.

Soon I would have to begin my preparations for the final medical and surgery examinations. Meanwhile I had some time to relax and take stock. My pleasures were to be found on the cricket field, in pubs, coffee houses and bookie offices, which led to occasional but necessary trips to the pawnbrokers. And there were the long conversations with other students about Ireland—about the Ireland that itself was being reborn. The National Theatre was in its early throes with Yeats, Shaw, Lady Gregory, O'Casey, Joyce its chief protagonists. The Irish language was being revived and Irish Literature became a recognized force in the world. My fellow students, particularly those from the rural areas, brought with them a fierce nationalism and a poetic idealism. They were engrossed with the importance of Ireland and her affairs and I, for one, did not wonder at its intensity. I cannot write about 'my medical school' without writing about 'my Dublin' for I lived there and experienced its pulsating throb of life, its timelessness and the magnanimity of its people.

True, Dublin life was not perfect. For instance, sex during my student life was a hazardous affair. In Dublin, contraception was a half whispered word. In rural Ireland there was a naive belief in the leprechaun magic of the anti-spermicidal effect of cigarette ends, brass wedding rings and pieces of coal. We, as students, sought continuously for the contraband which made the very thought of sex one of illegality and guilt. All that furtiveness! But there were many Nellies, Lilys, Carmels, Margarets, Marys and Bridgets in our lives, if not always in reality, always in the imagination.

However, the examinations of Medicine and Surgery loomed ominously and I had to engage in intensive book work and attend the clinics of the Dublin hospitals and the lectures of

Professor Abrahamson (The Abe) and Sir Arthur Chance who could so easily reduce in size patient and student alike.

At long last I completed the course, passing both examinations (I was awarded first prize and medal in Medicine). This was the day of days, or so it seemed to me then: my mother's telegram had arrived and the whole family were overjoyed. After all, each now yellowing message had heralded this day. Soon I would have to stand before the President of the College to swear the Hippocratic Oath. There they would sit, capped and gowned for the ceremony: Professor Jessop, Professor Abrahamson, Boxwell, Davidson, Evatt, Mr Stoney, Professor Micks and Sir Arthur Chance, and many other notable medical dignatories, climaxing as a frozen section the whole of my student career. It suddenly did not seem such a long time since my first success in obtaining entrance to the medical school or even since I had peered out of the window in Arnott Street at the cows and heard my mother's laugh. Yet it was hard to believe that I was now a doctor. It was said that I was the youngest student ever to qualify at the Royal College of Physicians and Surgeons. (I had to wait a number of months before I was old enough to be granted my license to practise.) Hymie Sharpe also had passed his exams and we celebrated our success together in Neary's pub, and then, to recuperate, by lying on the grass in the sun near the duckpond in St Stephen's Green, whence with our arms round each other's waist, we tottered unsteadily across the road to the solid block of the Royal College where the porter, Starkie, stood on the steps like a sentinel and said to us respectfully, 'Good evening, doctors.'

Edward Lowbury

Edward Lowbury was born in London in 1913. He went to St Paul's School and to University College, Oxford, where he held a medical scholarship and won two literary University prizes (the Newdigate and the Matthew Arnold Memorial). He took a degree in physiology at Oxford and completed his medical studies at the London Hospital Medical College. He trained as a bacteriologist at the Emergency Public Health Laboratory in Cambridge. After army service as a pathologist during the war, he joined the scientific staff of the Medical Research Council, for which he still works as Bacteriologist of the MRC Burns Unit at the Birmingham Accident Hospital and as Honorary Director of the Regional Health Service Infection Research Laboratory, which he opened in 1964.

He has published many papers and two books on medical and scientific subjects, nine books of poems, and (jointly) a book on Thomas Campion. He is a Fellow of two Royal Colleges (Physicians and Pathologists) and of the Royal Society of Literature. He is a Doctor of Medicine of Oxford University, and has been awarded an Honorary DSc by the University of Aston in Birmingham.

He is married to Alison, daughter of the poet Andrew Young, and has three daughters.

y father was a general practitioner in London. When I was very young he sometimes hinted that I might do worse than follow his example. The mysteries of his craft excited me, as when during an exceptionally long evening surgery my mother sent me to ask when father would be ready for supper, and he came to the surgery door transformed— wearing a laryngoscope mirror on his forehead; or when he spoke of an imminent 'confinement'. I was deeply interested in childbirth; even more than the proper wish to cure people of their illnesses, a craving to get to the bottom of this mystery about how babies arrive made me, at the age of nine or ten, decide to take up medicine.

There were snags. At school (St Paul's) I was on the classical side, and rather reluctantly moved across to science just when I was beginning to get something out of Latin and Greek; I was already hooked on English poetry and turning out imitations of Wordsworth and Milton. The change to science was traumatic. Out of my element, I was driven to despair when I heard my chemistry master advise a boy to pay at least as much attention to the notes as to the text of his Shakespeare set book for School Certificate; in retrospect, I think I probably misjudged that master. The storms passed, and after taking the necessary exams I found myself with a place at the Oxford Medical School and a narrow, top floor room at University

College ('Univ') with fascinating and time-consuming views—at one end onto the High Street, at the other end onto the main quadrangle of the College.

Pre-medical training at Oxford consisted of lectures and practical classes in the anatomy, physiology and biochemistry departments, backed up by a weekly physiology tutorial in College. In the third year everyone took an honours degree course, usually in physiology. In the fourth year some (I was one) stayed on for two more terms to attend an introductory course in pathology and to be initiated into clinical medicine at the Radcliffe Infirmary. A few, who had excelled in their honours degree course, stayed on to do research.

Morning lectures were often an anticlimax after the walk from College past the architectural marvels of Radcliffe Square and Parks Road, 'towery and leafy between towers'. If we were late at Dr Alice Carleton's anatomy lectures, she would politely but very firmly invite us down to the front row and then lay bare our ignorance with merciless quizzing; her erudition was immense, but it made students like myself, who had no talent for anatomy, despair of leaping that hurdle. In my second year Wilfred le Gros Clark took up the vacant chair of anatomy; with his ebullient, broad-jowled eloquence he injected a new spirit into the subject. A freshman's qualms on entering the dissecting room, however, were apt to be dispelled (though for some they were probably enhanced) by the irreverent and salacious humour of our old dissecting room attendant. The hours of dissection were strenuous, but pleasantly diversified by conversation between students sharing the remains of a leg or a brain.

I preferred the physiology course, and responded with enthusiasm to J. C. Eccles's lively discourses on the nerve impulse and on spinal reflexes. In this field the Oxford school was pre-eminent, through the pioneer researches of Sir Charles Sherrington and his team. Sherrington, who was in his seventies, still held the chair of physiology, and I attended some of his lectures. Though he was regarded by many as the greatest physiologist of his age, Sherrington was not a great lecturer, at least not to undergraduates, for whom his extreme caution in qualifying all statements blunted the impact of his words, and there were surprisingly few students in the large theatre where he lectured. I found it inspiring, though, to hear about an important branch of physiology from the man who had launched it.

During practical classes we had an opportunity of making personal contacts with some of our teachers. In the lecture room they might seem to have an Olympian omniscience, but when questioned in the classroom they would sometimes have no ready answer—a helpful insight into the limitations of knowledge, which was later reinforced by the degree course in physiology, when we learned that there were plenty of un-answered questions, and these might be the starting points for research. We, too, had questions fired at us, and our teachers sometimes lost patience with a student who persistently failed to answer or to answer correctly. I remember a recently appointed professor asking a tall, silent man in my year, 'What is a cholagogue?' (requiring the answer 'a substance that promotes the flow of bile'). When the student remained silent, the Prof snapped 'Think, man, think; what is a demagogue? What is a synagogue?'—to which the student responded slowly, with a mysterious smile, pointing a long finger at the seated master, 'What is a *pedagogue*!'

Once a week the medical students at Univ went, individually, for a physiology tutorial to our college tutor, Dr Ainley Walker, a short, elderly man with a bushy grey moustache, steel-rimmed spectacles, a kindly manner and a mischievous twinkle. Some-times, while I read my essay aloud, he would sit silent for quite a long time with his eyes shut. He was known, on such an occasion, to have stopped the reader with a grunt, saying 'Will you read those last few lines again; I was following a train of thought.' It seemed more likely that the student's voice had lulled him to sleep. My tutor gave me much valuable advice. He was concerned that I should waste no time, but recommended spare-time reading of good books, especially Trollope.

The range of recreation in Oxford was immense, and it was tempting for the student to spend most evenings at meetings, concerts, cinemas, and then to go on talking through the night. At the English Club I heard T. S. Eliot, Herbert Read, Edith Sitwell, W. H. Auden and the young Dylan Thomas talk and read their poems; I remember little that was said, but can still hear a cataract of word play from Dylan Thomas which ended with the phrase 'and there are fairies at the bottom of the guardsman'. At the Junior Scientific Club Julian Huxley, J. B. S. Haldane and many other famous scientists spoke to us. I heard Churchill speak at a political meeting in the Union about the dangers of German re-armament and saw a German student—an ardent Nazi—stamp out of the hall in anger. At our college we had a music club which arranged recitals by such artists as Solomon and Egon Petri; we also made our own music, and I particularly enjoyed musical evenings at the house of the Dean, John Maud (later Lord Redcliffe-Maud) and his pianist wife, Jean Hamilton. I belonged to a small club, The Martlets, consisting of twelve members who regarded themselves as intellectuals or aesthetes and read papers to each other on esoteric subjects. I did *not* belong to the Shakespeare Club at which the athletes and hearties enjoyed dinners, opened (so I was told) by the President proposing the standard resolution 'that the Bard be not read tonight'. After the dinner there was much tumultuous singing in the quad, and a closing of 'oaks' (the extra doors to students' rooms) by Martlets and others who feared invasion and broken windows.

On fine afternoons in the summer term I liked to take out a punt or a canoe on the Cherwell, usually with college friends, occasionally with a girl from St Hilda's; sometimes I took out a punt on my own, tied it up under a tree and tried (without much success) to read textbooks or papers. Many people spent the afternoon rowing or playing football or cricket. Others preferred to browse in the great bookshops on Broad Street. I had no talent for ball games (though I sometimes mishandled a bat or a racket); I can, however, record one unusual exploit on the playing field of Balliol. Having hooked a poetry prize at school, I decided to submit a poem for the famous Newdigate Prize; the subject was 'Fire', which seemed appropriate for a science student. One afternoon a newspaper reporter knocked at my door and told me that I had been awarded the prize (and forty years later, looking at the faded Blackwell publication of my 300-line effusion, I am stunned to think that such a beginner's effort caused quite a commotion, with press interviews and a *Times* third leader!). The winners of certain literary prizes, including the Newdigate, had to read passages from their compositions at the honorary degree ceremony (Encaenia) in the Sheldonian Theatre. We had a rehearsal in the empty Sheldonian on the day before the ceremony. I read my bit with what I took to be appropriate vigour, but when I had finished Cyril Bailey, the Public Orator, said he couldn't hear a word of it. He then led me to the playing field and told me to stand on the boundary, while he walked to the wicket. 'Now read your lines so that I can hear them,' he ordered; and after five or six failures I reached the required decibels. 'You must read like that tomorrow; and imagine that you are reading Shakespeare,' he added.

My tutor was worried by these literary antics, but pointed out that many Newdigate winners had gone on to lead useful lives as doctors, lawyers, scientists, politicians, etcetera. Dr Odgers, the fatherly Reader in Anatomy who habitually addressed us as 'my good man', said 'I should think you are a better anatomy student than Keats was'; and a brilliant zoology student, Peter Medawar, whom I sometimes met on visits to a mutual friend at Magdalen, pointed out that hardly any Newdigate winners went on to make the grade in poetry (Matthew Arnold was an exception). But though I wanted to become a writer, I had no intention of giving up medicine; indeed, it seemed to me that medical practice would be a better school for the would-be writer than literary studies, because books (I argued) are, or should be, made out of life, not out of books.

Nevertheless most of my college friends—Roy Lewis, John Penman, Maurice Wills and others—happened to be reading English, History, Classics and other arts subjects or non-medical sciences, and my own reading was mostly outside my curriculum. I lunched once a week with Edward Caldin, a chemistry student who had been a contemporary at St Paul's and shared with me a taste for philosophy. With Peter Crossley-Holland, one of my medical contemporaries, I escaped one morning from a biophysics practical class that wasn't going too well to have coffee at Elliston's and learn about Sibelius; Peter gave up medicine for music soon afterwards, and was for a time running music on the BBC Third Programme. I also came to know some of the non-medical dons. The one I remember best was C. S. Lewis, with whom I spent a June evening at Magdalen having an essay which I had submitted for a University prize gently torn to pieces. I think he was as much involved as I was, because it grew quite dark before he thought of switching on the light. What I learned that evening on the orderly presentation of an argument and the avoidance of verbal display was very helpful to me in the expression of scientific ideas as well as in 'creative' writing. Nothing, however, could help me.to catch up with the arrears of reading recommended by my finals tutor, Hugh Sinclair. I also had a lurking suspicion that physiology was not really my scene. Indeed, I was relieved to get a second in the finals.

While taking the physiology finals I became aware that Mr X, one of my fellow examinees, was suffering from paranoid symptoms. I had always known him as a quiet man with a puzzled expression, but now he was telling people that I had used hypnosis to drain him of knowledge which might have been useful to him but would now help me in the exam. When I returned to my digs after one of the papers, I was met at the door by my landlady who said, 'You had better not go to your room. A student has just been here, saying he'd like to see you.

He was carrying a knife. I didn't like the look of him. He said he would come back. . . .' From her description of his appearance I at once recognized Mr X. On the next day I noticed that X was not in the examination room, and I never saw him again.

During my third year I lodged in an ancient house in Holywell. I noticed one day that my landlady's housemaid, Dorothy, was looking unwell, with swollen glands in her neck. The next day I was told she was laid up with mumps. Soon afterwards I went down for the vacation, and returned next term to attend Professor Florey's excellent course in pathology and the introduction to clinical medicine at the Radcliffe Infirmary. This included attendance at some post-mortems. Through two years of anatomy I had acquired a certain detachment which enabled me to see a dead body as a structure and to focus, in the p.m. room, on the pathological changes. But when I recognized one of the bodies laid out for examination as that of Dorothy, disfigured by Hodgkin's Disease, my objectivity was shattered. For a time I wondered if I could stand up to the stresses of medical life. Later it struck me that a doctor needs a balance of objectivity and compassion, and that my shock on recognizing Dorothy was no bad response for one whose life was to be spent in caring for the sick.

In the summer of 1937 I left Oxford and entered the London Hospital Medical College to do my clinical studies. The newcomers were distributed in small groups to spend periods of three months attached to a medical or surgical 'firm', or in the Pathology Department, or doing midwifery, dermatology and other special subjects. On the clinical firms we were allocated patients whom we examined on admission and visited daily. We wrote detailed case notes and might be called upon to read them on the chief's teaching round. These rounds had a ceremonial character. Shortly before the hour at which the round was to begin, the 'clerks' or 'dressers' (as students on medical or surgical firms, respectively, were called) gathered under the clock near the main hospital entrance; the junior

resident (House Physician or Surgeon) took up his position
outside the chiefs' common-room, which was a little way along
the main corridor, and the senior resident (First Assistant)
knocked and entered the sanctum. Chief and First Assistant
would then emerge, the houseman would fall in behind them,
and the rabble of clerks or dressers would follow in an untidy
crocodile, racing to keep up if the chief happened to be Dr
Donald Hunter, moving more sedately behind Dr Russell
Brain or Mr Russell Howard. We entered the ward, were
joined by the Ward Sister and progressed from bed to bed,
the chief dividing his attention between patients and students,
and exercising his talents as diagnostician, comforter, educator,
wit and scientist. The style varied greatly with the personality
and character of the chief. Sometimes a patient was ruffled by
Dr Cox's passionate scientific interest in his illness, preferring
the kindly benevolence of the less scientific partner in the firm,
Dr Box; but another patient would say 'Give me Cox every
time; he really *knows* what's wrong with me.'

The personal oddities of our chiefs were a constant source of
entertainment at lectures, out-patient clinics and on ward
rounds; sometimes they helped to implant important medical
facts in our memory. I recall the first of Donald Hunter's
lectures on the anaemias, when he stormed into the lecture
room—lean, bald, bespectacled, with an agonized expression
and carrying a large open canister, which he suddenly jerked
upwards with great vigour; seconds later a hailstorm of small
pellets fell on our heads and desks, accompanied by the
thunder of Hunter's voice roaring 'Blaud's pills! Now you will
understand why it's unpardonable to prescribe such stuff for
patients when there are quite palatable alternatives.' Hectic,
aquiline and full of gesture, Hunter delivered his lectures with
a passionate intensity, an abundance of brilliantly defined
examples and a richness of wit and irony. The more hilarious
his utterances, the more serious—even pained—became his
expression. He was sometimes provoked by wrong answers to
outbursts of fury. 'Your ignorance,' I once heard him bark, 'is

encyclopaedic.' Another time, when a student could not answer the question 'How does one prepare Vitamin D?' Hunter said, with an air of breathless excitement, 'Well, let me help you', and led him down the garden path with a patently absurd description of the process, in the manner of Heath-Robinson. 'O.K.?' 'Yes, sir'; and then from Hunter, wringing the culprit's neck, 'You great boob!' followed by an unforgettably precise account of the process. From Donald Hunter I first learned, through practice, the notion of a normal 'control' when he sent me to the X-ray department to borrow the film of a healthy femur to compare with one of a femur that seemed to show some clinical abnormality.

We had lectures on tropical medicine from Dr Manson-Bahr, a robust personality who enlivened his discourse with reminiscences of medical practice in tropical countries. I was charmed by the account of his weekly out-patient clinic in, I believe, Cairo. Patients who had had dysentery were asked to bring a specimen of faeces with them to these clinics for laboratory examination. People used a great variety of containers for their specimens. One day he asked a patient why he had not brought a specimen, and the man replied 'I *did* bring a specimen, and it was in a sardine tin; but someone sitting next to me in the bus stole it from my pocket, and I didn't have the heart to say "Give that back!" '

A surgical teacher whom no 'Londoner' of the nineteen-thirties could ever forget was Russell Howard. He was a heavy, elderly man with a slight stoop, a scowl, a plebeian twang and a lively directness of expression. He would glare through a monocle attached to a ribbon while waiting for a student to answer a question; when the answer provoked or surprised him, the eyebrows went up and the monocle fell dramatically from his eye. He was a stickler for punctuality. 'You're late, Mr Fletcher,' he snapped as a student came into the lecture room. 'Detained at stool, sir,' chirped Fletcher; to which R.H. fired back 'Well, Mr Fletcher, since surgical out-patients I bin and 'ad tea with Sister Gloucester *and* passed me water and got 'ere in time.'* He often shot questions on anatomy at us, and complained of our ignorance. 'And where's Poupart's Junction?' Someone started 'Where the inguinal ligament . . .' but was cut short with a stentorian 'Nonsense; it's about a mile out from Waterloo Station!' And so it is.

Dr Russell Brain, the distinguished neurologist who was also a connoisseur of literature and the arts, could be disturbingly silent. He did not respond to social chatter, and gave the impression of not wishing to speak unless he had something significant to say. His manner was gentle but austere. I was his house physician soon after I qualified, and remember lunching with him in almost complete silence; then suddenly he spoke, with enthusiasm, of the novel by Henry James which he was reading, and said the writing of James shared some qualities with that of Proust. When he was at Oxford he had known the famous Dr Spooner, who spoonerized his name to 'Brainy Russell' (or was it 'Rainy Brussell'?). The only time I have either used a leech or seen one used was on one of Brain's patients, at his suggestion; the method was once so common that doctors were sometimes called 'leeches'. Though famous for his silences, Brain gave us beautifully articulated clinical lectures and commentaries, as did that other neurologist, George Riddoch, in his attractive Aberdonian lilt; Riddoch seemed to address all his male patients over fifty as 'Daddy' and all the rest as 'Laddy'.

Dr Clark Kennedy, the Dean, was a memorable personality, tall and lean, with a wide expressive mouth and the air of a king-sized hobgoblin; the pre-Christmas revels presented him convincingly as 'Dr Dark Remedy'. I was impressed by his words to newcomers on the importance of compassion in our contacts with people who were suffering the worst of human hardships. His manner of lecturing and questioning was friendly, even paternal, with a certain smiling solemnity. Once, while

---

*I was recently reminded of this episode, which I half remembered, by my contemporary and friend, Ronald Henson.

talking about focal sepsis, he pointed to a student and said 'If you were a bacillus, where would you choose to live?' The student was non-plussed, but a voice from another row was half-heard to mutter 'The Dorchester.'

These and a number of other teachers left an enduring impression. So did some of the students. Oddly, the first student to do so was one whom I mistook for a teacher—a distinguished-looking middle-aged man wearing a bow tie and pince-nez with a black ribbon. I was flattered when this character brought me a fresh sheet of paper while I was taking notes at a post mortem for the pathologist, Billy Woods, but soon realized the situation when Woods began asking him a few questions about pathology. It appeared that he was one of those permanent students who repeatedly failed their qualifying examinations because, so it was said, they had been left a legacy 'to cover the period of medical studies'. At the other extreme were those students who sailed with ease through exams while leading an apparently carefree social life. No doubt they were equipped with excellent memories. To most of us the amount of knowledge that had to be absorbed was formidable. As I travelled by underground each day to and from my parents' house in Hampstead (nearly two hours of travel), I did not have the opportunity of getting to know any of my fellow students well, though later, when I was a resident, some whose acquaintance I had made while we were students became friends.

Another group of people whose presence influenced our lives in various ways were the nurses. There were the stern, senior sisters—'dragons' who kept order in their wards by sharpness of command; one of these sisters stands out in my memory, a small, fiery creature with the voice of a sergeant-major whom we called Pixie, but feared. Others with gentler ways seemed to keep as good a discipline in their wards. And there were attractive staff nurses and probationers whose presence made the night round, when we were residents, a happy occasion, with tea and whispered conversation. The moral welfare of the nurses was carefully guarded, and no male was allowed into the Nurses' Home except, on conducted tours, during the annual garden party. Once, when I was a junior house physician, a ward maid called Susie, whose behaviour had caused some concern, brandished a bottle of lysol in sister's face and said she would kill herself by drinking it. Susie was admitted for observation to the medical ward on the second floor where I worked. While I was writing up case notes in the ward one afternoon I heard two or three patients call out; they were telling me that the patient in bed 3 had gone out of the ward on to the fire escape. Susie's bed was empty. I dashed out to the fire escape. Half way down the iron staircase was Susie, her white nightie blowing in the wind. I followed at top speed. Susie dashed across the courtyard and straight into the Nurses' Home. She may have imagined she would be safe against male pursuit in this female preserve, but I followed her through the door, and up the staircase. Her energies were flagging, and I caught up with her on the first landing. She refused to walk, so I carried her down the stairs, and noticed, with some satisfaction, one of the most ferocious of the sisters standing at the foot of the stairs—and thinking, no doubt, that I was abducting one of her night nurses. I greeted the sister politely, and received, in reply, a look of icy stupefaction but, to my surprise, no words. She may have doubted the evidence of her senses. Later that day Susie tricked a nurse, who was attending to her in the bathroom, to fetch something from the ward, and immediately locked herself in. She then climbed on to the window ledge and threatened to throw herself down, but eventually yielded quietly to the entreaties of a little crowd below and went with 'the gentleman' to another hospital for special treatment.

There was a flourishing dramatic society at the Medical College; I heard Russell Howard complain that a student's memory was much better at learning his lines than at mastering his surgery. During one season the Society put on a production of J. B. Priestley's *I have been here before*. The producer thought it would be a good idea to invite Bernard Shaw to attend the premiere, and sent him an invitation card, which came back inscribed 'Unluckily (for you) I have, G.B.S.' Dramatic talent sometimes extended into other spheres. I passed the telephone in the lobby of the students' 'Athenaeum' one day and saw a droll contemporary of mine, called, I believe, Ramsbottom, carrying on a long conversation in which he kept changing the timbre of his voice. We soon found out that on lifting the receiver Ramsbottom had heard the caller say 'Is that Liverpool Street Station?' and promptly answered 'Yes.' The caller then said he had a load of machinery that he wished to have delivered to Harwich by train, 'I'll put you through to the Goods Department,' said Ramsbottom and then, with a new voice, 'Goods Department.' The caller repeated his request. 'I'll have to ask the Manager,' said 'Goods Department'; and the poor caller repeated his request in response to at least four different voices, all emanating from the same throat. I often wonder what happened to that machinery—and to the wicked but resourceful Ramsbottom.

When we were doing midwifery we lived in accommodation near the hospital, ready to be called at any moment to attend deliveries in the labour wards and, for part of the time, in patients' homes on the District. It was a happy time, because for the most part we saw healthy women and helped them to perform a normal function. Almost always there was a jubilant atmosphere after the birth, even in the poorest houses. On receiving a call I went to the 'patient's' home with an experienced midwife, who addressed me as 'doctor' (for that is what I was taken to be). One of my fellow students was accosted by the drunken husband of a woman in labour. 'What's this I hear,' he said, 'about students being sent out on the District? If I saw a student comin' to see my wife I'd give 'im somethink to remember.' And then his eyes brightened as a thought struck him; 'Ere, are *you* a student?' My friend protested convincingly that he was not, and no bones were broken. Work in the District was sometimes done under difficult conditions, and I remember attending a delivery by candle light, as there was no electricity.

During the midwifery period I first heard an unholy sound which we later came to know as the air-raid warning siren; it was a trial sounding. The probability of war began to dawn upon us. When it came, the wards were made ready to receive casualties, and there were now better opportunities for general clinical experience outside London; so during the three months before my medical finals I returned to the Radcliffe Infirmary in Oxford, which had now become greatly enriched by the generosity of Lord Nuffield. After a door-to-door hunt for digs, I found a convenient room in St John Street, where my land-lady looked almost exactly like my former landlady in Museum Road. I was beginning to wonder about the influence of occupation on facial contours when I discovered that the two landladies were sisters! My own sister had just started her first term at Somerville College, and I sometimes had a bath there, as the geyser in my lodgings delivered either a very small amount of hot or a normal volume of tepid water. It was strangely calm and harmonious, a sunlit, mellow season which I remember with peculiar pleasure, in spite of the war and the imminence of my exam.

After qualifying we were, technically, doctors, but our studies continued while we held resident and trainee appointments. In my case, a stick of bombs falling on Mile End Hospital, where I was house surgeon in September 1940, made it necessary for me to move on to a fever hospital. The clinical experience there of infectious diseases prompted me to apply for a bacteriology traineeship in the Emergency Public Health Laboratory at Cambridge. I was accepted. One morning, not long after my arrival, I was examining cultures of diphtheria bacilli, when an elderly gentleman with flowing grey hair, a bow tie and remarkable eyes walked in and asked for the Director. I told him that Dr Downie was out but would soon be back. The visitor stayed and wanted to see what I was looking at, so I showed him the cultures and explained, in layman's language, the differences between different types of diphtheria bacilli. 'I'm in the same line as you,'said the visitor, and at that moment Dr Downie came in and said 'I see you have met; this' (to the visitor) 'is Lowbury who has just joined us; and' (to me) 'this is Professor Alexander Fleming.' My embarrassment could not have been greater if I had known about penicillin which, in 1941, was still known only to cognoscenti. Many years later, as a member of an MRC Committee on antibiotics, I came to know Fleming well enough to realize that I need not have been embarrassed. After Cambridge the road led, via pathology appointments in the Army, to work for the Medical Research Council. Excited by the new medicine which had developed during and after my student days, I was drawn into the field of antibiotic research which Fleming and Florey had pioneered, but it was the accident of a bomb which drew me away from clinical practice. As a writer I was a bit alarmed at this turn of events, but soon discovered a new argument for wearing two hats, for I had noticed that there was some common ground between the practice of scientific research and the writing of poetry—in hitting upon useful ideas and expressing the ideas and the experimental results in living language.

My two medical schools were, in many ways, complementary. The teaching I received in the physiology course at Oxford emphasized the growing points and gaps in knowledge, the disciplines of research and the critical reading of original papers. At the London Hospital the approach was more dogmatic, and the unwary might have imagined that all knowledge was wrapped up in their textbooks and lecture notes. Paradoxically, this air of certainty went with the exercise of much diagnostic 'art' and some more or less inspired guesswork. On the social side, Oxford gave the student, fresh from school, a bewildering range of experiences and an environment of great beauty and antiquity, but with residues of monasticism; the effect could be unsettling as well as enriching. At the London Hospital the student, more mature when he entered the wards, was surrounded by patients whose suffering and disability contrasted with his own well-being, and evoked compassion, resilience and humour. I had the impression that psychological disturbance was commoner among students at Oxford than at the London; but perhaps this was just matter of growing up.

Patrick Trevor-Roper

Patrick Trevor-Roper was born in 1916, and was educated at Charter-house, Cambridge and Westminster Medical School. He spent three war years in Italy with the New Zealand Medical Corps, and was appointed Consultant Eye Surgeon at Westminster Hospital in 1947, then at Moorfields and King Edward VII Hospital.

He has published a number of books on ophthalmology, and also about art and music; and for over thirty years has been editor of The Transactions of the Ophthalmological Societies UK. *He is President-elect of the Ophthalmic Section of the Royal Society of Medicine, and was granted in 1977 its first De Lancey Award 'for furtherance of the link between art and medicine'. He is also a founder member of the International Academy of Ophthalmology.*

As Adviser to the Royal Commonwealth Society for the Blind, he has made professional visits to underdeveloped countries nearly every year, running mobile eye units, founding an eye hospital in Addis Ababa, and opening one in Lagos during the Nigerian Civil War. His elder brother is Regius Professor of History at Oxford.

I became a medical student because we lived over my father's surgery, and it seemed the natural thing to do.

He was born in 1885, a fourteenth child. His father's tuberculous leg evidently curtailed the series, and in my father's only memory of him, he was being carried upstairs, past all the tearful children, to have it sawn off on the kitchen table, which had been placed alongside their newly-installed bath. My grandmother then married his cousin, another Trevor-Roper, but he too died soon afterwards, and my father remained the youngest. From infancy he had crippling asthma, which could only be allayed by drinking 'Vinum Ipecachuanae', relieving the spasm by making him vomit. This was concocted from cheap sherry, so that he could never drink sherry during the ninety-odd years that have followed. As a severe asthmatic, he was rejected by the Indian Medical Service because of his poor life-expectancy; so, in 1910, he bought a practice near the Scottish border for three hundred pounds, and has remained there ever since, a kindly sceptic, an admirable (if, in early years, a rather remote) parent, and until his recent retirement, an excellent GP.

My decision to do medicine was easy, but pre-war Charterhouse was not a school which lightly encouraged boys to lapse into fringe subjects like biology, and I was constrained to plod on with Latin and Greek until I had gained a Senior Classical

Scholarship, before I was let off the hook. My brother, Hugh, two years my senior, was by then the light of the classical sixth, and I (visibly less talented) was the more expendable. He moved on to Oxford, and I applied to Cambridge, not really to escape from his shadow but because our science masters all came from Cambridge and suggested no alternative.

Biology had many rewards. We could go on 'nature rambles' and escape the exquisite tedium of those long cricket afternoons, standing far out in the field, knowing that every daydream would be punctured by a missed catch, or waiting endlessly in case called on to bat (only rarely could one retreat into the long grass, for romantic moments among the tall buttercups). I almost looked forward to the winters with their action-packed fifty minutes of soccer; and even volunteered for an experimental rugger team—the helter-skelter was fun, but whenever it got exciting the whistle seemed to bring it all to a halt. Along with biology, and an escape from parading with the OTC, these last years at school seemed designed to expunge the often brutish memories of the first; even the liberal doses of chapel were not without appeal to an emotional and rather indrawn adolescent such as I was.

The transition to Cambridge was inevitably abrupt. The freedom and the surroundings (particularly at Clare) were delicious, but many of us in those slow-maturing days missed the breast-feeding of our organized schools; we would willingly have savoured some interesting vices if only we had known where to find them. It was accepted that girls were hard to get to grips with: there were only a few town tarts (most of us were far too timid) and odd Girton girls we met at lectures who bicycled back to their fortress well before dark. This left us with a few emancipated Newnhamites who were on an easy seller's market. I finally took one of these to a May Ball and other dates followed, but she was very buttoned-up. Indeed she retired to an asylum shortly afterwards!

So, rather by default, when we male students tired of talking and listening to music, we capitulated to our formidable lecture list, and that kept most of us out of mischief. Everyone was political then; and, since most of my friends were socialists, that seemed a good enough reason to become a devout conservative. This was quickly reversed when I moved to Westminster Medical School, where a conservative orthodoxy was universal. I have remained at Westminster virtually ever since, and some radical attitudes have even survived the damaging Barbara Castle epoch.

In retrospect my Cambridge period was agreeable and unadventurous, except for that spirited summer vacation of 1936 when I and a fellow student bought horses in Budapest, and rode eastwards into Czechoslovakia, finally selling them at a village auction. But patches of gloom and tedium are easily overlooked, and the events of those three years now seem to have been enacted in a sepia-tinted haze, set against the background of bells and chiming clocks and the smell of new-mown grass.

By 1937 I was ready to move on, and selected Westminster Medical School because its entrance scholarship happened to be the earliest in the London list, and I was prepared to work my way through the lot. I knew even then that Small was Good, but the poky little house in Caxton Street that served as Westminster Medical School rather overstretched this general truth. When I saw the hospital, a great Gothic palace confronting the Abbey Sanctuary, I knew that all would be well.

Westminster Hospital was founded in 1715; the first of our voluntary hospitals. Until then London had been served only by the great mediaeval foundations of St Thomas in Southwark and St Bartholomew in Smithfield, which posed a difficult journey for those who lived and ailed under the shadow of Westminster Abbey, in the marshes of the 'Islet of Thorns' between the arms of the Tybourne delta. In 1720, its first establishment was opened on the corner of Petty France (where it was replaced by the dismal block of Queen Anne's Mansions, and later by Sir Basil Spence's even greater monstrosity), and within a few yards of the house in which the blind John Milton had dictated the last cantos of his *Paradise Lost*. Then, after several short hops, it reached the west front of Westminster Abbey, where it swelled like a large broody hen to dominate the whole precinct.

I remember my first weeks at Westminster Hospital. A wide flight of steps led to the great front doors, and on into a cathedral-like vestibule. At its far end a broad staircase swept upwards to lead into the entrance of a chapel, from whose stained-glass window, over the distant altar, blue light filtered down into the vestibule. At the chapel doors the stairs divided, to curve around the side walls as a balcony, and meet again in front at the entrance of a majestic board-room. Inside that vestibule, as in an opera setting, everything seemed to be happening. Little processions wound to and fro, led by a venerable consultant, followed by his registrar, his houseman, and a troupe of students, all in white, with their stethoscopes dangling; only the croziers were lacking. Patients, almoners, officials, friends and hangers-on all drifted about, as in a market place. Occasionally bodies on stretchers would be carried in, sometimes decently covered by a pall (on one occasion, the drapes concealed two bodies, sheepishly linked in vaginismus); and they would pass on to the adjacent 'Casualty', another huge room filled with humanity. There, in the seats around its walls, were patients having their ears syringed, wounds dressed and so on. So that the stretchers, being deposited on two central tables and there unveiled, provided a welcome diversion for all. At the great front door stood a time-battered notice that all bags must be open for inspection—to catch any bottles of gin being smuggled in to the patients.

That central vestibule was the hub of hospital life, and even the most timid of new students felt that he was being welcomed into a rich and varied community.

There was no briefing for the neophyte, nothing resembling our present introductory courses. One plunged straight in. My first lecture in the adjacent medical school was by coincidence given by the oculist I was destined to succeed, A. F. MacCallan, and he opened it by displaying on our old epidiascope the frontispiece of the book he had written on Trachoma, showing a bust of himself, in glory outside the hospital in Cairo that he had founded. Some weeks later Sir Stanley Woodward opened his lecture by producing a gold 'demi-hunter' watch from his waistcoat pocket, declaring that this was the first requisite for a doctor, since it inspired confidence; the rest of his lecture discussed the virtues of the different European spas.

After this lecture came the ward-round. I had been allocated to the firm of our then Senior Physician, Hildred Carlill, a quasi-neurologist, who practised rather elementary hypnosis on many of his patients, in the main quite successfully, although often for rather bizarre reasons ('Now repeat "I must not have intercourse with my wife while she is pregnant"; now once again "I must not ————" '); he also, like Shaw's Cutler Walpole, firmly believed in the 'nuciform sac' as the cause of most ills (if he inserted his long forefinger, and pressed hard into the right pelvis, he could nearly always elicit some appendicular tenderness). It was a formidable start to clinical medicine, but not very arduous since a third of our patients were spending weeks under Somnifane narcosis (hoping to remedy their habit-spasms and so on), and another third were mourning the loss of their (apparently sound) appendices. Carlill, I soon discovered, had more idiosyncrasies than most of his fellow consultants, to whom he was often rather an embarrassment. Indeed on one occasion he was sued by a female patient, whose limp he reckoned was hysterical, for forcing her to demonstrate her gait, stripped to the panties, in front of the boardroom. But in those days, high-handed eccentricities were expected of the more senior consultants who, since they were unpaid for their services, were very hard to discipline or control. Indeed, Carlill's predecessor, Sir James Purves-Stewart, was even less inhibited: he processed through his wards like a bishop followed by his house-surgeon bearing a gold patella hammer, then a secretary ready to record his comments, then his chauffeur carrying the box of other instruments, and then his disciples. At the end of his career he proclaimed that he had found a vaccine for multiple sclerosis, and the queue of wretched sufferers stretched daily into the abbey sanctuary, waiting for the miracle cure. When the treatment was exposed, Sir James retired to the safe isolation of a lighthouse on the Sussex coast, and was never seen again at Westminster.

The hospital was controlled by a Board of Governors, a set of grandees, who, as far as we were aware, were irrelevant and infinitely remote; but their secretary, the wise and efficient Charles Power, evidently administered the show almost single-handed, along with his able and helpful treasurer, E. S. Gower. Nowadays, the administrators have proliferated like paramecia and even outnumber the medical staff; they all have prolix and unrememberable titles, and shift jobs so often within the vast hierarchy that personal contact is hard to achieve; only Charles Power's successor, Patrick MacMahon, who now presides over the maelstrom, provides reassurance and continuity.

The old hospital building was a glorious Victorian extravagance but the old medical school was appalling. There was only one seedy common-room, with horse-hair settees, faintly smelling of stale beer and tobacco, and a primitive lecture room, with steeply rising tiers of hard, narrow benches that smacked of the Middle Ages. The Dean, Sir Adolphe Abrahams, was sartorially perfect, and rarely seen, and his secretary we avoided. But upstairs was 'the Pathology', run by Professor Pulvertaft ('Bulgey', because of his slight exophthalmos), helped only by his Registrar, Magnus Haines and by Joe Humble, his Houseman. These did all the work which now keeps forty doctors (including five professors) busy. Pulvertaft gave us delightful lectures every morning, and wrote gentle poetry in the evenings. Magnus and Joe patiently showed us how to assess the test-tube samples and gobbets of human anatomy we brought along, like young retrievers, every morning.

It is difficult at this distance to recapture the excitement and trepidation which attended my first bedside encounters. Even the simplest blood-letting became a major enterprise, and the surface anatomy I had learnt from corpses became even more alarming when I was called on to explore the most intimate regions of a body that was not only sentient, but often a bundle of apprehensions. It was hard to retain that initial façade of confidence as I hunted for an elusive spleen, squeezing away on the naked abdomen of someone I had never seen before, who, whether timid, truculent or just bored, inevitably knew that I was only small fry. And it was weeks before I could, with nonchalance, lift up a dependent breast to tap the chest wall beneath, or invaginate a scrotum with my forefinger to define an inguinal hernia, or any other of those immodest excursions which were soon to become commonplace. My own emotions were so often further wrenched when the patient recited her troubles and I guessed what was amiss, and realized that one morning I might find her silent and cold in the bed.

Cultural activities in the medical school were restricted to an annual 'Beer and Smoker', in keeping with the bleak squalor of the common-room in which it was held. And at weekends the more energetic of us travelled many miles to a sports ground in the suburbs. Nowadays we have an Arts Festival which takes over the Medical School for ten days each summer, a thriving orchestra, drama and film societies and so on. And we still win the rugger cup as well. I had left a Cambridge in which the Spanish war, rearmament, Hitler and the Oxford group dominated discussion. Inside Westminster Medical School the outside world seemed barely to exist, politics were rarely mentioned, unorthodox views scorned. In retrospect it was a grubby, Philistine, self-centred universe. Perhaps I do it an injustice, but the school had been at a low ebb for some years, even 'reduced' to accepting women students from 1916 to 1929 for lack of male applicants, and only the prospect of the new buildings gave it the transfusion it needed.

Then came the war. Both hospital and medical school had moved in the nick of time to our new site behind the Abbey— with buildings which, although architecturally undistinguished, were spacious and well-lit. They gazed at each other across the old graveyard of St John's in Smith Square, and were linked by a tunnel which passed between the corpses; their vast lower basements reposed comfortably on the gravel bed of the old delta, encased in water-proof asphalt. Attached to the medical school was the new nurses' home; and each linking corridor was barred by a locked door. Fire regulations required the key to be available in a vulnerable glass-fronted box—a gift to the more spirited students and a constant despair to the matron. Recent matrons have abandoned the struggle; access is free.

My first two war years were largely spent within the confines of our new hospital and medical school, as a resident student and then house-physician. In that curiously enclosed world a corporate life emerged; we turned to each other for company, and no longer hurried off from the medical school as soon as possible each day to join outside friends, who generally came from the equally enclosed university world we had relinquished. Now, with travel difficult, and, by the second winter, with air-raids starting before the day's work was done, we were back in a resident community, enhanced by the handful of con-sultants and registrars who had joined us, as an 'Emergency Medical Service' team, ready to cope with the war casualties.

Westminster had already become more attractive to potential students, as the new buildings emerged, for only one other London teaching hospital, Middlesex, had been rebuilt during the century, and that on a pattern barely distinguishable from its Victorian predecessors. The presence of a bar in our common-room (an unprecedented concession) and the accessi-bility of nurses may have helped. The quality of our student-life was already looking up by the beginning of the war—annual pantomimes, annual formal dinners, a music society, a reconstructed student magazine, and so on. We have never looked back.

Of course there were travails. Three bombs hit the hospital, and one of them trapped me in the lift, but fortunately while the door was still open. A second bomb later tipped the operating table and patient into the joint laps of the Eye Surgeon and myself while we were busy digging débris from his damaged cornea.

This surgeon, the junior eye consultant, who happened to occupy the next mattress to me in the underground locker-room, where we all clustered overnight, turned out to be an ideal companion, sharing my pleasure in opera and owning a quantity of '78 records with which to while away the time. I had never realized that surgeons could be so civilized. Through the eyes of a student, at any rate, successful surgeons had all seemed to be rumbustious, Philistine extroverts, sometimes butchers, sometimes masterly technicians, but with no time for arts or abstractions. So, dazzled by the sensitivity and taste of my neighbour, I slid into being an ophthalmologist, and moved on from Westminster to become house-surgeon at Moorfields. There, from a chance remark across the operating table, I gathered that one of my predecessors had got into trouble in the Middle East and was being hurried home to New Zealand. So I shyly offered myself at New Zealand House as his replacement; and was enlisted forthwith. Wearing my new boy-scout hat and puggaree (which I later discovered had been abandoned by their expeditionary force many years previously), I had soon embarked.

I was still in Italy, with the New Zealand division, when Germany collapsed, and had already acquired a primer in Japanese, anticipating a leisurely journey to the Far East, followed by demobilization in New Zealand; and after that my well-trodden daydreams led on to anywhere but home. Then Hiroshima was bombed, my daydreams vanished, and I drifted back to London. I had become a doctor to emulate my father, and an ophthalmologist because I wanted to emulate the sympathetic surgeon whom chance had placed beside me in our air-raid shelter. So the following year, I gravitated back to his clinic at Westminster, and have contentedly occupied the same stool in our Eye Department ever since.

Sheila Sherlock

Sheila Sherlock was educated at Folkestone County School for Girls and Edinburgh University, where she graduated in 1941. She was awarded the Ettles Scholarship as the most distinguished student of the year and a gold medal for her MD thesis. After graduation she worked under the late Sir James Learmonth in the Department of Surgery in Edinburgh and proceeded to the Postgraduate Medical School of London (Hammersmith Hospital) where she studied under Sir John McMichael and the late Professor E. P. Sharpey-Schafer. She was lecturer and Honorary Consultant Physician at Hammersmith Hospital 1948–1959.

A Rockefeller Travelling Fellowship allowed a period to be spent in the Department of Physiological Chemistry at Yale University. Staff appointments have been at the Postgraduate Medical School and since 1959, Chairman and Professor of Medicine in the Department of Medicine, Royal Free Hospital, London, where she is honorary Consultant Physician. Research interests have been in all aspects of the liver as applied to disease in man. She has written numerous papers and a textbook, Diseases of the Liver and Biliary System *(1955), now in its 5th edition, and widely translated.*

She is a Fellow of the Royal College of Physicians of London (Vice President and Senior Censor, 1976–77), a Fellow of the Royal College of Physicians, Edinburgh, and an honorary Fellow of the American College of Physicians and the Royal Canadian College of Physicians. She is also an honorary Fellow of the Gastroenterological Associations of Australasia, Mexico, and Costa Rica, and is a past President of the British Society of Gastroenterology and of the International Association for the Study of the Liver. She sits on the Senate of the University of London. She is an honorary D.Sc. of the City University of New York.

Professor Sherlock is married to Dr D. Geraint James, Dean of the Royal Northern Hospital, London, and they have two daughters.

The Edinburgh Faculty of Medicine was founded in 1726, soon to be followed in 1729 by the opening of the Royal Infirmary, at about the same time as Guy's Hospital (1725), the London Hospital (1741) and Middlesex Hospital (1745) in London. I spent six happy years in this medical school and look back with affection and with pride to my time there.

My journey from London to Edinburgh was by road in a coach without the benefit of the M1. It was October 1st, 1936, and I was arriving in Edinburgh to start my medical training at the University. My adrenalin was turned on both from excitement and travel sickness as I climbed the Mound to spend my first night in a Church of Scotland women's hostel. I had only been accepted for medical training on the 15th of August. The past year had been a series of frustrations and interviews for admittance to medical school. I had been rejected everywhere. I had even studied St Mark's Gospel in order to take a theology entrance examination at King's College, London, but was unsuccessful. It was even more difficult for women to enter medicine then than it is now. I shall never know what factor determined my late acceptance at Edinburgh University. Certainly, I could pull no strings. This late acceptance has coloured my feelings towards Edinburgh, both then and now, and accounts for the rather rosy glasses with which I have, in later life, viewed the training received and the personalities I encountered.

The emphasis in the pre-clinical years was the Edinburgh tradition—anatomy, with much learning by heart. Men and women students dissected dessicated human bodies in separate rooms. Mixed dissecting was somehow indecent, although these mummified remains provided a completely asexual atmosphere. Our teacher was E. B. Jamieson, a taciturn man from the Shetlands. He wore a black skull-cap, smoked a large hooked pipe, and kept his distance from the women students. He gave one lecture for men students only. It was said to cover the facts of life, but I doubt if he knew them. His splendid anatomy textbooks were republished every year and reached out to medical students throughout the world.

Physicians helped to teach both anatomy and physiology. Surgical registrars came over from the Infirmary in the afternoons to help in the dissecting rooms. Junior physicians took the practical physiology classes. My chief-to-be, Sir John McMichael, was in charge of the bicycle ergometer, and J. D. S. Cameron, later President of the Royal College of Physicians of Edinburgh, taught us the physiology of the nervous system. He emphasized the importance of the simple pin in neurological examination and scorned more complicated procedures. Ninian Bruce used to draw the parts of the brain on the blackboard, two hands simultaneously. He was ragged unmercifully, the elegant performance taking place to a background of chiming alarm clocks and cock-crows. With the present shortage of medically-qualified teachers in pre-clinical departments of medical schools, it always amazes me that clinical teachers are not integrated more into the basic science curriculum as they were in my Edinburgh. Their influence on the pre-clinical student is profound, longlasting and practical.

Teachers took tremendous pains in preparing their material, even for informal bedside demonstrations. The lack of such preparation surprised me greatly when I encountered clinical teaching in London medical schools. Here Consultants often walked casually in for their teaching rounds hoping for the best. In Edinburgh, teaching took priority over all activities, except medical emergencies.

Jimmy (Poppa) Learmonth, the Professor of Surgery, was my favourite teacher. A highly intelligent man, he exemplified the best of Scottish academics. He had reached the Chair of Surgery in Edinburgh via research into the nerve supply of the bladder at the Mayo Clinic and the Regius Chair of Surgery at Aberdeen. Every teaching session he gave had been carefully thought out and was accompanied by a typewritten handout summarizing the facts. Neat, tidy, quick-tempered and with a biting tongue, he frightened some students, but others adored him. I idolized him. He was extremely punctilious, and banished students who were just three minutes late at the door of the lecture theatre. He used white gloves when drawing on the blackboard as his skin was reputedly sensitive to chalk. He was to become a Royal for he performed a lumbar sympathectomy on King George VI. When driving past Buckingham Palace he proudly pointed out the room where the operation had taken place. The juniors selected for his support always regarded him as 'Poppa', and he behaved as such. When I was engaged to be married, he came down on the night train from Edinburgh, inspected my fiancé over breakfast at King's Cross Hotel, and then returned home. When my first-born arrived he was quickly on the scene, presenting me with a grouse's foot for good luck. We remained friends until he died in 1967 from cancer of the lung. He had been a very heavy smoker.

The late John Fraser was an outstanding teacher and surgical operator. He could always be relied upon to put on a good teaching show on Wednesday mornings in Ward 3. His acolytes stood by making sure he demonstrated the right patient, or operated on the right side or indeed the right organ, for sometimes he was carried away by the tempo of his performance.

The most thoughtful surgeon was Ian Aird who was then about to go off to the war. I was to know him far better when we were both colleagues at the Postgraduate Medical School, London (Hammersmith Hospital) after the war. In 1939, he was making ends meet by running a cram course for young surgeons who were hoping to pass the Fellowship of the Edinburgh College of Surgeons. His notes for this course were in great demand during the war and fetched enormous sums on the black market. Later, they formed the basis of his celebrated *Companion of Surgical Studies* which appeared in 1949, and which has been continually revised and lives today. He was a pioneer of transplant surgery who wrote, 'Perhaps the future lies in the surgery of replacement . . . There are however still basic biological problems of enormous complexity concerned with protein chemistry, genetic, and even the primary philosophical problem of individuality which bars us from the transplantation of even such relatively simple material as skin from one individual to another.' These prophetic words must have been written in the early 1960s.

Aird's most famous operation at Hammersmith was the separation of the Nigerian Siamese twins, Boko and Komu. In spite of his achievements as teacher and investigator, particularly as head of a world-famous department of surgery, he always doubted his own surgical technical abilities. His end was a tragic one. Gripped by severe depression, he commandeered an enormous dose of barbiturate, ostensibly for surgical research, from a Hammersmith Hospital dispensary. A true Scot, he refused to pay the two shillings Health Service dispensing fee. He then retired to the doctors' quarters and did what he felt had to be done with the efficiency expected of him. His farewell reflected his upbringing as the son of a Calvinist mother and former President of the Edinburgh University Christian Union: by his bedside was a Bible open at Ecclesiastes, Chapter 3—'Vanity of vanities, saith the Preacher, vanity of vanities, all is vanity.'

Stanley Davidson was our Professor of Medicine. He had

helped to overcome leptospirosis in Aberdeen herring cutters.
He is an outstanding haematologist and his lecture notes
formed the basis of the internationally-acclaimed Edinburgh
textbook of medicine (Davidson and Dunlop). He had a
reputation for 'counting the bawbees'. Nevertheless, when he
retired, he donated the whole of his superannuation monies, a
not inconsiderable sum, to the University of Edinburgh, and
has since made numerous, very generous gifts, both to the
University and to the Royal College of Physicians of Edinburgh.

Derrick Dunlop was the Professor of Therapeutics. He
taught every Wednesday afternoon, a voluntary course, but
one which attracted packed lecture theatres. He was dark and
even more handsome than Stanley. I can see him now, pacing
up and down the theatre, lisping to us about the 'woad to
Uwaemia' and the fate of kidney patients in those days. Apart
from the book he wrote with Professor Davidson, he had
written his own *Textbook of Therapeutics*.

D. K. Henderson was our Professor of Psychiatry. He had
received his formative psychiatric training at the Johns Hopkins
University in Baltimore, and was an organic psychiatrist
opposed to Freudian analysis. He was also the author of the
current standard textbook on psychiatry. His weekly out-
patient clinics were a revelation. Patients were interviewed in
a lecture theatre with an audience of a hundred students, yet
such was his rapport with the patients, that he could discuss
intimate details of their personal life freely and without their
objecting. In fact, they seemed to benefit from 'getting it off
their chest' in front of an audience.

These teachers of ours found the time and had the ability to
write textbooks which kept the name of the Edinburgh Medical
School evergreen in medical schools around the world. They
deserved their international awards of merit.

The Edinburgh graduate was trained up to a wide knowledge
of medicine, because each specialty had its own little examination, from which there was no escape. Nobody could sit his
finals until he had collected a pack of DP (duly performed)

certificates in each side specialty. This diversity has helped me considerably when faced with conditions outside my own particular field of interest. Medical students, particularly in the United States, specialize too early and miss a lot of the fun of the fair. In my Edinburgh days, attendance at a lecture was recorded by handing a signed white visiting card to the janitor at the door of the lecture theatre. There was a bit of cheating, of course, if a friend was capable of palming multiple cards. The majority of lectures had been conscientiously prepared and many were superlative. I still believe in the lecture system as providing a firm basis for medical education. The brilliant student may find it unnecessary, but it is valuable for the dull, ordinary and lazy ones, and more important at that stage than an hour at bridge, billiards or under the hairdryer.

Today's so-called 'new' medical curricula emphasize repeated in-course assessments of students by mini-tests and teacher evaluation. This differs little from the old Edinburgh system of the 1930s and 1940s with its many class examinations and 'duly performed the work of the class' certificates at the end of each assignment.

We university students shared teaching facilities in the Infirmary with those from the Royal College of Surgeons (Surgeons Hall). These students were largely from the United States, Jews from New York City who had failed to be accepted in their own medical schools. A similar problem exists for Americans today. The old Surgeons Hall is no longer an undergraduate medical school and its role has been taken over by such universities as Bologna, Geneva and Padua, and by Guadalaquira in Mexico. The American students were older than we were. They lived in groups in small apartments and cooked themselves exciting kosher meals. They lived on a shoe-string and like their counterparts today, worked very hard. They were always to be seen with large specialist textbooks under their arm, tomes we did not know existed. During the long summer vacation, they returned home to become firemen in New York or waiters in New Jersey, or garage hands in

Boston. This provided the means to continue in Edinburgh for another year. (They have since become distinguished physicians and surgeons in the United States and are proud of their Edinburgh connections.)

I too had to work during the summer holidays. In the long vacation of the pre-clinical years, I returned to Folkestone, and worked as a waitress in the local Tatler tea-rooms. It must have been a horrific performance. I also worked part-time as a tutor in Basil Paterson's cramming school in Palmerston Road. I taught physics, chemistry, and mathematics to candidates for the Scottish highers and for university entrance. This was useful training for my later career as a university teacher.

The Edinburgh Union adjoins the new quadrangle where medical teaching takes place, and abutts the MacEwen Hall. It served as a social centre in a non-residential University and was a substitute for Oxford and Cambridge colleges. And like most of them, it did not recognize women. An exception was made on Saturday nights, when it became a fun dance-hall Palais, so they had to have women. We danced the Veleta, the Gay Gordons, the Dashing White Sergeant, and I wore a long blue taffeta gown. The gay bucks of the Union leant against the walls drinking beer and lamenting the lack of talent. Afterwards, we went to the foot of the Mound, where a coffee-stall sold bacon rolls—a real treat in the days of wartime rationing.

The Women's Union, on the other hand, was rather prissy and jolly hockeysticks. I did not join, for the same reason that I have never joined the Medical Women's Federation. Women in medicine, and indeed in any other profession, must advance on merit and not because they are fighting as an under-privileged minority. If a woman is intelligent and is determined to apply herself then she can reach the top nowadays without the help of women's organizations. What is more important is to choose a sympathetic, understanding husband.

The Cosmopolitan Club was my favourite club. It was held on Sunday evenings, always a dead time in Edinburgh. It took place in the home of Dr G. B. Ludlam, a Senior Lecturer in

Zoology, and a Quaker. The Ludlam family allowed their home to be invaded every Sunday by upwards of a hundred students from all over the world to hear subjects of general interest. I well recall Stephen Spender reading his poems. The President was David Pitt, now Lord Pitt, Chairman of the Race Relations Board. A Jamaican, he qualified in medicine in Edinburgh and later went into general practice in East London. He was also the President of the Edinburgh Students Representative Council.

Even with a war on, the cultural life of Edinburgh continued. The theatre was particularly flourishing, with previews of many of the shows which were to be successes on the London stage, and with gallery seats at the Kings Theatre costing only sixpence. I remember John Gielgud in *Love for Love* and Edith Evans in Shaw's *Heartbreak House*. Coward's *Design for Living* with Anton Walbrook, Rex Harrison and Diana Wynyard opened up a sophisticated new world for me. Mother had never explained a ménage à trois. Donald Tovey held the Reid Chair of Music and kept us happy at the Saturday afternoon Reid concerts which he conducted.

The traditional Edinburgh University student was a local, or near local boy or girl, who had attended one of the large secondary schools such as George Watsons, Heriots, or Stewarts. These schools are the pride of Edinburgh, and the students from them had come up to the University to get a degree and to get qualified, come what may, and that was the end of it. The men were on the whole mannerless and with narrow views. They despised women medical students heartily and I suppose, in retrospect, we did seem a pretty drab lot. These 'native' students lived at home, and what allegiance they had was to their old school rather than to the University. They attended classes on a nine-to-five basis and took little part in any extra-curricular activity. They were on the whole hard-working and certainly raised academic standards. They played tennis, hockey and rugby for their FP (former pupil) school teams rather than the University. This selection did, and probably still does, markedly lower the standard of university sports. Others from further afield in Scotland and elsewhere lived in lodgings. There were plenty of these all over Marchmont, Warrender Park Road, and thereabouts. They cost £1.50 to £2 a week with breakfast and high tea and with full board on Saturdays and Sundays. It is said that the Royal Navy tradition depended on 'the Grace of God and its petty officers'. Edinburgh medical life would substitute in the maxim 'its landladies'. For this sum of money, some of them also acted as counsellor, psychiatrist, priest or guru. A Highland minister and his wife unexpectedly arrived in Marchmont Street late one night and called at the lodgings of their student son. The father rang the bell and somewhat uncertainly enquired, 'Is this where Mr MacDougall lives?' 'Aye,' replied the landlady with forlorn resignation. 'Carry him in. His bedroom is up the stair, first on the right.'

There were only one or two Oxford and Cambridge graduates, mostly those who had a Scottish family background and wished to return home for their clinical years. Their time at Oxbridge had made them much more worldly-wise, and they were excellent students. One of them, A. A. Guild (BA Cantab), was one of the best students in my year. He eventually worked as Superintendent of Lambeth Hospital but died too young, from primary liver cancer following hepatitis he had acquired during Army Service. There were also a few Sassennachs like me.

My best friend was Esther Davidson, who came from a large academic Edinburgh family. She was always slightly 'fey', extremely absent-minded, and disorganized with appointments, dress and even her way of life. On graduation, she trained for, and became, not surprisingly, a psychiatrist. From then on, she did brilliant work in London, and on alcoholism in the ghettos of New Jersey. Sadly, she developed a pre-senile dementia in her early fifties and for the last years of her life she was virtually a vegetable. After her death, her devoted mother collected the poems she had written during her life

and published them privately. This is an outstanding anthology
of her views on people and life and the cities she had known. I
recommend it to doctors and patients alike. This poem was
written when she was a medical student:

> Shall these bones live?
>
> *I am like a desert sand*
> *Where no oasis is,*
> *A parched and sterile land.*
>
> *I who have held the brand*
> *Of unquenched fire*
> *Whose flames the poets fanned.*
>
> *Disbanded is the choir,*
> *Unpractised is the hand,*
> *Unsung the lyre,*
>
> *Between my temples spanned*
> *A vacant lot for hire*
> *Where hyacinths may stand.*

I had little money to spare in my student days. My mother
and I lived on a £60 per annum grant from the Kent Education
Committee (£30 of this was a loan!). My old school, Folkestone
County School, gave me a scholarship of £120 per year. With
the money raised from vacation jobs, this had to cover living,
books, tuition and examination fees. I recently came across an
old account book showing how the money went. Many books
had to be bought at that time and these were usually obtained
second-hand. Among them were such classics as Hutchinson
and Hunter's *Clinical Methods*, Boyd's *Pathology*, Clark's *Pharmacology*, Mackie and MacCarthy's *Bacteriology*, and Muir's
Atlas of Pathology. A. J. Clark and T. Mackie were of course our
teachers. *Aids to Medicine* was always in my pocket. The
matriculation fee to the University was compulsory and allowed
participation in most student activities. A hospital ticket

permitting practice in the wards of the Royal Infirmary *in perpetuo* cost £18. My old account book contains other interesting items such as Year Dinner—two shillings; tennis team photo—three shillings and sixpence; golf clubs—four shillings; broken slide—one shilling. A hilarious obstetric course, spent at the National Hospital, Dublin, cost £16 (the fare being only £2.14s, and the subsistence for two weeks £5.16s). My teacher in Dublin was Eammon De Valera, the late President of Eire's son.

Finally, on July 6th, 1941, we all graduated. The morning started with a visit, clad in hired academic robes, to the photographers. (My portrait shows me looking slightly self-satisfied.) The Graduation Ceremonial took place in the MacEwen Hall, an enormous edifice built on brewing profits and rather like the Albert Hall in miniature. Cockerels are released from the balconies at the time of Rectorial elections. On this occasion things were more peaceful. D. K. Henderson gave the address. He took his text from John Buchan, 'Patience shuffle the cards'. As an impetuous Aries-born, I often think of it. Over the years, this text has stood me in good stead. In the evening we had a ball at the New Cavendish Dance Hall. I can remember little of it.

In a couple of days, I was off to Perth to do a locum tenens in general practice—pre-registration House Physician and House Surgeon appointments were not compulsory then, before one was set loose on the world. I was substituting for Dr Grace McRorey, who was going on holiday. She had a very general practice. I rode around Perth on a bicycle, visiting the patients, and in her office, collected half-crowns from those who could afford to pay them. Wives and children were not eligible for free medical care. Two weeks were enough to convince me that the rest of my life was not going to be spent in general practice.

My mother, who had nourished me throughout my training, was delighted when I landed the Ettles Scholarship, awarded to the first of the year. I was the second woman in the history of the Medical School to receive this award, so they did not have much experience of coping with feminist problems. The Ettles Scholarship would normally open the doors wide to plum House appointments at the Royal Infirmary, but not for a woman at that time. The Residency was a sacred male precinct, but perhaps they had no toilet facilities for women. Poppa Learmonth overcame the impasse by appointing me to an academic post as an Assistant Lecturer in Surgery. I was virtually a House Surgeon assisting at operations, but even at that stage, I had an opportunity of becoming interested in medical research. Poppa taught me how to organize results, how to write a paper, how to review the scientific literature. This I have passed on from perfectionist Poppa to my junior colleagues over the years. At the end of the year, Poppa begged me to give up surgery. I had snipped too many pairs of his operating gloves. But he paved my way to an academic future by arranging for my transfer to Hammersmith Hospital to work under another Ettles scholar, the great Sir John Mc-Michael, FRS.

I went to Edinburgh in 1936, an impecunious Kent County student. In the subsequent five years that I was a student there, the University gave me a bitterly cold climate, warm friendship, a place in the Edinburgh University Tennis Team, outstanding teaching, and a road to a future in academic medicine. These are rewards enough for any young girl.

Dannie Abse

Besides being a doctor Dannie Abse is one of Britain's leading poets. In 1947, while still a medical student at Westminster Hospital, he had his first play produced and, not long after, his first book of poems was published. He also began working on Ash on a Young Man's Sleeve, *a novel about his youth in South Wales which now has become a set book in schools and a modern classic. A year after qualifying he served in the RAF, achieving the rank of Squadron Leader. On de-mobilization, he was appointed by Air Vice-Marshal Sir Aubrey Rumball, the chief RAF medical consultant at that time, the civilian physician in charge of the RAF chest clinic at the Central Medical Establishment in London.*

In 1956, he became medical correspondent to a Sunday newspaper, continuing however with his clinical chest work until 1973 when he was invited to the USA to be the Visiting Senior Fellow in Humanities at Princeton University. On his return to the UK he has continued his dual career of doctor and writer, the progress of which he relates in his autobiography A Poet in the Family *(1974). In 1976 his most recent play,* Pythagoras *was produced at the Birmingham Repertory Theatre, and last year his much acclaimed* Collected Poems 1948–1976 *was published in the UK and in the USA.*

alf the family are doctors. There is my eldest brother
Wilfred, my father's brother Max, my mother's brother
Joe. There are my two Ammanford cousins and also
two other cousins from Cardiff, Michael and Jack. So when
the family meets on those rare ceremonial occasions of celebra-
tion or lament, it is less a family gathering than a medical
conference.

In 1937, when I, a small boy, said, 'I wouldn't mind being
a vet'—the cat lay motionless on its cushion on the carpet, its
electric eyes staring at nothing and would not sip even a little
of the warm milk I was offering it—my brother Wilfred said
masterfully that I might as well become, like so many others
in the family, a doctor. 'Sick people,' he maintained with the
authority of one who had read *Twelve Great Philosophers*, 'are
more important than sick animals.' I stared unhappily at the
cat while my father, overhearing our conversation, teased,
'You think this duffer has enough intelligence to become a
doctor?' My eldest brother replied without irony, 'All you
need is average intelligence to become a doctor. He'll manage
it. We ought to think seriously about putting his name down
for the new Westminster Hospital Medical School that they
are planning.'

My mother used to say, 'Dannie never thinks of tomorrow.'
She was wrong. I did and I do. But I rarely think of the day

after tomorrow. That is why, perhaps, I have always resisted the idea of buying Life Insurance and that is certainly why, also, that since the question of what-are-you-going-to-be-when-you-grow-up had been solved, I thought more of being a medical student than a doctor.

Wilfred had only just qualified. For years I had heard about medical student experiences and pranks. Had not Wilfred cured a baffling case of hysterical blindness through hypnosis? (Wilfred was going to be a psychiatrist.) And only eighteen months earlier Wilfred had been doing his midwifery and the telephone had sounded *after midnight*. That's how important it was to be a medical student.

True, on that occasion, Wilfred had to go to a house in Zinc Street to deliver a baby. The voice commanding him to do so had, apparently, been Welsh and urgent and hoarse. So my big brother, hero Wilfred, with his little black bag, climbed on to his bicycle and made for Splott. He did not know that Mr and Mrs Jones of Zinc Street had only just married, were still on their blissful honeymoon, and had no immediate plans to have a baby. He did not know that the hoarse, urgent, Welsh voice was that of another medical student conning him.

It was raining in the district of Roath, Cardiff, where we lived then and from where Wilfred set out, and it was raining in the district of Splott, Cardiff, when he arrived on his bicycle, flustered and damp, at a dark door in Zinc Street. Clutching his little black bag he banged at the front door till a light went on upstairs, then a light in the hall, and finally the door opened to a sleepy, burly, tall lock-forward in pyjamas asking, 'Mmm?'

'Where's your wife, Mr Jones?' asked Wilfred.

'Upstairs in bed,' replied the burly man, surprised.

And he was even more surprised when Wilfred said, 'Good,' as he pushed past him and ran up the stairs enthusiastically.

Yes, I thought, it may be fun to become a medical student, to mess around like that, and save every now and then one or two lives! I fancied myself walking down Queen Street with a stethoscope sticking, like a credential, out of my pocket.

Some years later, in 1941, during my last year in school when I was studying those pre-medical subjects, biology, chemistry and physics, I was to hear much more about the crises and practical jokes of 'med' students. Three of my friends—a year older than I—were already at the Welsh National School of Medicine. When I joined them at their Students' Union to play poker they were full of medical gossip: how Spud Taylor after a rectal examination on a woman had diagnosed, to the delight of all the other students, an enlarged prostate; better still, how Tonker Davies had cut off a penis from one of the cadavers in the Anatomy Room, put it in his trouser pocket before going to a student dance and, eventually, when the last waltz was being played—'Any umbrellas, any umberellas, don't mind the rain'—Tonker had pulled it out of his trousers much to the consternation of his partner!

Such was the tenor of the conversations of these friends of mine, these first-year medical students. Their talk was frequently anecdotal in that way, bawdy or about sport. They were never philosophical while sober. As the record turned on the Medical Students' Union radiogram and Dinah Shore sang 'Body and Soul' or 'Smoke Gets in Your Eyes' or 'Sophisticated Lady' I never heard any of those poker players vulnerably say why he wanted to become a doctor or confess to aspirations of doing good in the world. They pondered on nothing more awesome than a Royal Flush. Or so it seemed. As for me, though I was beginning to write poetry (I was told it was 'just a phase'), I felt happy in the company of such friends. I certainly did not feel like the composer Berlioz who had written, 'Become a doctor! Study anatomy! dissect! witness horrible operations ... Forsake the empyrean for the dreary realities of earth! the immortal angels of poetry and love and their inspired songs for filthy hospitals, dreadful medical students ...'

No, I wanted to become one of those dreadful medical students myself. My regret was that I could not stay at home and study at the Welsh National School of Medicine. Finally, though, I did not so much leave home as home left me! For, during a February air raid (the night turned luminous green because of flares), it seemed some German pilot mistook Roath Park Lake for Cardiff Docks and bomb after bomb whistled down to cause explosions followed by lonely silences. The house next door disappeared and part of our house collapsed. Injured, I was taken to Bridgend Cottage Hospital where I was looked after by one of my Ammanford cousins. 'Look after this boy,' he kept winking at the nurses, 'he's valuable, he's going to become a doctor.'

Nineteen months later, in September—that month of cool suggestions and pleasant sunlight a shade too yellow—I arrived in wartime London, the train doors in Paddington Station banging behind me like gunshot reports. My cases made my arms long for they contained not only predictable contents but my brother's weighty medical textbooks and the half skeleton he had bequeathed me.

These I unpacked in a boarding-house room in Swiss Cottage. I put the femur, tibia, the armbones, the wired foot, the wired hand and the skull in the wardrobe and the textbooks—on the flyleaf of each was written, D. Wilfred Abse, *Nil Desperandum*—on the mantelpiece. I was ready 'to go', ready to begin my studies at King's College in the Strand where Westminster Hospital students, along with those from Charing Cross Hospital, King's College Hospital and St George's Hospital, spent their pre-clinical years.

King's College in the Strand was cold, shabby, capacious and murky. It sounded of footsteps on linoleum and stone. Even when no one was about, the place sounded of ghosts in slippers. It smelt of stone and the nineteenth century. Because of air raids, most students, other than the medics, had been evacuated to provincial cities, so it was more obviously empty, stony, murky than ever. My first ordeal was to firewatch on the roof of King's one moonless night when the air raid siren had sounded. The second ordeal, a daytime one, was to enter the Anatomy Dissecting Room and to be assigned one half of a male body.

The formalin that preserves the cadavers pricks the eyes and has a reeking odour that seeps insidiously, pervasively, into one's clothes. And the cadavers themselves seemed so helpless and naked! Still I did not bolt as Berlioz had done in his day. 'Robert,' wrote Berlioz, 'asked me to accompany him to the Dissecting Room at the Hospital de la Pitié. When I entered that fearful charnel-house, littered with fragments of limbs, and saw the ghastly faces and cloven heads, the bloody cesspools in which we stood, with its reeking atmosphere, the swarms of sparrows fighting for scrapings and rats in the corners gnawing bleeding vertebrae, such a feeling of horror possessed me that I leapt out of the window as though Death and all his hideous crew were at my heels.'

Revulsion does not endure. I remember how, a few weeks after the commencement of our anatomy course, I observed one student, who earlier had been particularly fastidious, drop his lit cigarette accidentally into the open cavity of a dead abdomen; then, unthinkingly, he picked his cigarette up, put it back in his mouth, and went on dissecting with no sense of disquiet or disgust. The medical student soon forgets that the body he is dissecting was once alive. It becomes a model. Later I was to learn, during my clinical years, the live patient in the same way would often become a 'case'.

I did not enjoy anatomy; it was a chore to commit to memory the coloured plates of the Anatomy Book, to recall in detail, and as clearly as an eidetic image, the Rembrandt painting one had made for oneself by laying bare muscles, tendons, arteries and nerves of a body that gradually became smaller and smaller as it was dissected away. That I had to spend so many hours in the Anatomy room, that students everywhere had to learn in minute detail the anatomy of the human body (and embryology) seemed ridiculous to me. By the time we qualified most of us would have forgotten all but the most important details. Now I know that this cloudy remembrance of the subject makes us no worse doctors, for the knowledge we acquired so obsessively, and at such pains, and that we lost with such felicity, is quite useless for the most part in the general practice of medicine. Even those, who, as postgraduates, specialize in surgery, have to relearn the subject.

It amuses me, as I write this, to try and remember the vessels and nerves close to the ankle—I have worked in a chest clinic for years—but all I can recall is the mnemonic that helped me once to pass a viva: *Please Don't Vaseline Nellie's Hair*. The 'V', I suppose, stood for one vein or another and Nellie for a nerve the name of which, at present, I cannot recall.

I preferred the Physiology lectures. Professor MacDowell entertained us. 'We have three instincts,' he would say, 'three instincts, gentlemen. One could call them the three Fs: Fear, Food and Reproduction.' It seemed Professor MacDowell would sometimes be consulted by patients concerned about their hearts. But that year, for reasons of wartime economy, the lifts at King's were not working and the Professor's office was high, high up, close to the roof. Thus the heart patients had to climb all those endless stone steps.

'I don't have to examine them when they reach my door,' he said. 'If they make it that proves their hearts are sound; if not, then it's just a question of writing out the death certificate.'

In the early summer of 1944 I took my Anatomy and Physiology examinations. I passed them and so at last entered Westminster Hospital where I could wear a white coat with a stethoscope sticking out of its pocket. It was the time of the doodlebugs and suddenly there I was in the Casualty Department, hopelessly at a loss, while some stricken woman, lacerated to pieces by flying glass, was lifted from a stretcher in great pain and just kept on saying over and over, 'Oh God, oh dear, oh God, oh dear, oh dear, oh dear, oh God.'

I wonder how many medical students during the war had a sense of guilt. I had sometimes. My brother Wilfred was in the Army in India, and my brother Leo in the RAF in Egypt. My cousin Sidney had been killed at Dunkirk. All my old friends, other than medical students, were in the Services except those few who had already died 'pro patria'. In some ways one's vague sense of guilt in being allowed to complete one's studies was mitigated by working unnecessarily long hours in Casualty, assisting the harrassed doctors even if it was only by putting in stitches and bandaging, by tapping hydroceles, or giving gas and oxygen anaesthetics.

One afternoon, escaping from Casualty, I attended Psychiatric Outpatients. Wilfred in a letter had suggested, 'Make yourself known to Dr Ewing whom I know quite well.' But that afternoon another psychiatrist was taking Outpatients. He had a strong Viennese accent, a most reassuring thing in a psychiatrist, and he seemed pleased to see me. In fact he was enthusiastic. 'You can take Outpatients yourself,' he beamed. 'You've come just in time.' Startled, I explained that I had only been at Westminster Hospital three weeks or so and did not feel capable of taking on any Outpatients, never mind psychiatric ones. 'I haf to be somevere at three,' he said. 'It is good. And don't vorry, you know how to take a case history, yes? Zen take a case history and zen tell them to return next week ven I vill see them myself.' Even as I was objecting he was racing for the door shouting, 'Nurse! Nurse!'

So, wearing a white coat, I sat behind a desk like a real doctor and the nurse sent in the first patient for me to see. My very own first patient. I knew how to take a case history. Only a week earlier I had been taught that in Casualty. First you had to put down *Complaining of*, and then you asked the patient, 'What are you complaining of?' and the patient would say, 'I have a pain here in my left chest, doctor, that comes on after exercise.' And so you would write that down opposite *Complaining of*. It was quite simple really. Then there were other headings such as *Past History, Present History* and so on. Easy as winking.

Except my first patient complained of his wife. 'She gets up in the middle of the night,' he told me, 'because she reckons she hears voices. Then she walks up and down, walks up and down for hours and hours. I can't stand it.' After listening to his grumbles, inspired, I said, 'Now, I want you to bring your wife here next week and then we'll sort things out.' To my horror he replied, 'But she's outside, doctor. She's come along with me.' It was evident that I had to see her so, swallowing, I nodded and said, 'Then I'll see her right away. Would you mind waiting outside?'

His wife baffled me. She complained of her husband. 'He says he hears voices and gets up in the middle of the night and walks up and down remorselessly for hours. I can't bear it,' she said.

I did not know which one was crazy, who was hallucinating, which one was telling the truth. On her case history sheet I wrote 'complaining of her husband's strange insomnia' and on his case history sheet I wrote 'complaining of his wife's strange insomnia.' And the following week I never came back when they came back and I avoided that Viennese doctor ever after. The great thing was they both had called me 'doctor'. Neither of them called me 'sonny'.

In the autumn I joined my first medical firm and attended Ward Rounds. A dozen white-coated students on the firm would accompany the white-coated consultant physician, his white-coated registrar, his white-coated house physician, into the ward where sister and nurses fussed next to the beds of those patients who were to be examined and demonstrated to us. The consultant would walk two inches above the parquet floors unaided while the rest of us laughed at his quips, fawned, nodded wonderfully at aphorisms. 'One finger in the throat and one in the rectum makes a good diagnostician,' the consultant said quoting Sir William Osler, and some of us remembered another saying of Osler's which was, 'Look wise, say nothing, and grunt.' I often had to grunt when cross-examined on ward rounds.

Occasionally I would identify too much with the patient. I remember frequently worrying as we withdrew to the corner of a ward to discuss Mr Brown's symptoms that he, over there, half supine in bed, staring at us, would overhear low voices muttering 'malignant' or 'progressive'. However kind, consultants were not invariably tactful.

Indeed, on one occasion, as we stood around the bed of a patient whose history had been related to us in detail, I was asked to hazard a diagnosis. 'A duodenal ulcer,' I suggested. The patient smiled at me benignly. The consultant shook his head. 'No, Mr Green hasn't a duodenal ulcer. He has a chronic gastritis. You need to have some intelligence to have a duodenal ulcer, don't you, Mr Green?' Mr Green laughed— perhaps it was the laughter of contained aggression, I don't know. But he laughed and the students laughed a second later, so did the house physician, and the registrar, and the consultant most of all. 'Yes,' said the consultant, patting Mr Green's shoulder as if he were a good boy. 'Ha ha ha. You're lucky. You're too stupid to have an ulcer.' As we walked towards the next patient I looked back. Mr Green's head lay on the pillow. His eyes were closed.

A few weeks later, one afternoon while the firm waited for that same consultant who for some reason that day had been delayed, his registrar decided to teach us a singularly important principle of medicine. He asked a nurse to fetch him a sample of urine. He then talked to us about diabetes mellitus. '*Diabetes*,' he said, 'is a Greek name; but the Romans noticed that bees liked the urine of diabetics so they added the word *mellitus* which means sweet as honey. Well, as you know, you may find sugar in the urine of a diabetic . . .' By now the nurse had returned with a sample of urine which the registrar promptly held up like a trophy. We stared at that straw-coloured fluid as if we had never seen such a thing before. The registrar then startled us. He dipped a finger boldly into the urine then licked that finger with the tip of his tongue. As if tasting wine he opened and closed his lips rapidly. Could he perhaps detect a faint taste of sugar? The sample was passed on to us for an opinion. We all dipped a finger into the fluid, all of us foolishly licked that finger. 'Now,' said the registrar grinning, 'you have learnt the first principle of diagnosis. I mean the power of observation.' We were baffled. We stood near the sluice room outside the ward and, in the distance, some anonymous patient was explosively coughing. 'You see, ' the registrar continued triumphantly, 'I dipped my *middle* finger into the urine but licked my *index* finger—not like you chaps.'

Apart from ward rounds, I also attended lectures. I do not know now, objectively, whether they were tedious and badly presented, or whether it was simply that I was a poor listener. But Dr Ernie Lloyd's introductory lecture I found memorable. I did not know, then, that he delivered this same lecture in the same way every year. Ernie could have been a stage Welshman. He looked more like Lloyd George than Lloyd George did, and certainly he was just as histrionic.

He began in his sing-song accent, 'Today I shall talk to you about the heart, the old heart. It beats, do you see, seventy, duw, eighty times a minute; minute in, minute out; hour in, hour out; week in, week out; month in, month out; year in, year out. The old heart.' And as his incantation continued he used his hands like a conductor and as if we, his audience, were a silent orchestra. I hear his voice still: 'And the sound, oh the sound of a mitral murmur, it is like, oh aye, it is like . . . the wind; the wind rustlin' gently through the corn. [Long pause] Po-etic, isn't it, boys?' At Outpatients, I learned many things from him—also 'facts' that later I was to discover were quite wrong—for instance, that pulmonary tuberculosis never affected the right middle lobe. Well, I also learnt that there never was any 'never' in medicine.

There were many other Welshmen besides Ernie Lloyd at Westminster, not least C. Price Thomas, a brilliant chest surgeon (who was to operate on King George VI) and who, having visited the USA before the war exchanged his Welsh accent for a strange Yankee one. Drawling, he would address each student as 'Professor'. Touching his glasses he would ask some timid student, 'Why do you think that, Professor?' Many of the students themselves were Welsh. On one notable occasion so many of the cricket XI were from Wales that when we went out to field our captain gave us his orders in Welsh. The opposing side called us Welshminster.

In 1945 I joined my first surgical firm. It was always a question of doing things for the first time: first time to take blood from a vein, first lumbar puncture, first major operation, first post mortem, first childbirth, first death of a patient one had attended in the ward. Only repetition can lead to confidence so all these first times were a strain. No wonder so many medical students are frivolous. They are seldom mature enough to cope with so much ineluctable human sadness and sickness. What can young men and women do but make jokes, laugh and respond by some form of activism—in one mood horseplay, in another by trying to comfort and give help to those in the sick wards they so timidly linger in?

The most radical surgeon at Westminster Hospital was Sir Stanford Cade. How many times did I, along with other students on the firm, hear him conclude a graphic description of a patient's disease with the decision, 'This is inoperable.' And then, after a pause, 'I will operate.' One student on the firm at that time was 'Charlie' Westbury who was to become Sir Stanford's most brilliant pupil. Today Charlie gives those same ward rounds at Westminster Hospital and he, too, has become a radical surgeon, one universally respected.

Recently I met Charlie again. He startled me. He said that he had read a poem of mine called 'The Case' and wished to take issue with the suggestion advanced in the poem—that doctors, too often, see patients not as rounded human beings but simply as cases. (My poem was about a physician who knew the electrocardiograph of a patient but not the patient's name.)

'You see,' Charlie continued, 'if I saw some of my patients as rounded human beings and not as cases, because of the distressful nature of the surgery I have to undertake—sometimes in severely ill, pathetic children—I wouldn't be able to function. Give me so many inches of anonymous skin under the lights in an operating theatre and then I can use my skill; but if I were in a street and someone was knocked down then I'd find it difficult to cope.'

So much then for the so-called extroverted, tough personality of surgeons. Charlie was sensitive as a student and he is sensitive now. All the same, I do not think he found his student days, with their blatant confrontations with suffering, such a testing time as I did. The medical student learns more than the art and practice of medicine. He learns something about himself—and this is so whether he studies at Westminster Hospital, the Welsh National School of Medicine or Timbuctoo.

For my part, I found myself more and more given to reactive though purposeful daydreaming. For instance, I would be in the post-mortem room and as the pathologist was trying to teach us morbid truths about diseased tissues I would not hear what he said as I kept thinking how the mesenteric colours inside the exposed abdomen resembled those of a cathedral window; or at Outpatients or on a ward round I would find myself trying to write a poem in my head. Mr MacNab, on one ward round, woke me up, I remember. The rest of the firm were all staring at me. Evidently I had been asked a question. They waited. Mr MacNab waited. 'Your name is Abse,' he said sarcastically. 'This is Wednesday afternoon, this is the Westminster Hospital, Christmas is coming and it is 1946.'

In fact the consultants at Westminster were amazingly patient with me. Earlier, in June 1946, my first book of poems was accepted for publication by Hutchinson so perhaps they expected a budding poet to be somewhat disarrayed.

I was more than disarrayed. For the next eight months I hardly attended Westminster Hospital and in the summer of 1947 I returned to Cardiff where I pronounced to my brothers that I no longer wished to become a doctor, I wanted to become a writer. I had a book coming out, some of my stuff was being published in periodicals, I had also written a play. 'You can't give up medicine,' Leo said angrily. 'Father has made many sacrifices so that you can study in London.' Wilfred agreed and added forcefully, 'It will be better for you—I tell you so as a psychiatrist—to finish something that you've begun. If you don't it will mark you for the rest of your life. Besides, if you knuckle down you could qualify in a year. Then you could do what you like. Become a free-lance writer if that's what you want—*after you've qualified.*'

It took me more than a year to qualify but I am glad that after a further six months absence from medical school I eventually took their advice. When I did return to the wards again, continuously, seriously, I must have been intensely self-righteous and smug. For I had decided that one must act purely, selflessly! In order to do so, I argued, one must live like a patient recovering from a serious illness. One must always be grateful—for a grateful man is more likely to bear gifts to others. I would take the skull out of the wardrobe to help me in my meditations. I discovered, then, with exalted melancholy, that the skull ceased to be an anatomical artifact but truly a skull and a reminder of my own destiny. It became a threat, a sacred object that could help me extend my consciousness. I wanted to achieve lucidity and to act only with awareness. For some months a number of patients at Westminster Hospital had to endure my over-enthusiastic acts of kindness.

Two years later, when I, a doctor, returned to Cardiff to take on a general practice locum for my Uncle Max, I was not only aware of my own inadequacies but also the inadequacies of my medical education. I no longer stared at a skull and indeed rarely thought of the skull beneath the flesh. Worse, I understood the truth and shame

> *Of motives late revealed, and the awareness*
> *of things ill done and done to others' harm*
> *Which once I took for exercise of virtue.*
> *Then fool's approval stings and honour stains.*

But such introspection was time-consuming and, perhaps, self-indulgent. A voice on the 'phone was saying plaintively, 'Doctor, please, doctor.'

Michael O'Donnell

I'd constructed the question carefully in the bar of The Two Sawyers before crossing Lambeth Palace Road to the Dean's Office.

'Could this hospital entertain the idea of a part-time medical student?'

'Is there any other kind?' asked Allen Crockford, secretary to the Dean.

I'd reached his presence via a Part One in the Cambridge Natural Sciences Tripos, a Part Two in the Footlights and a spell in repertory that convinced me that I'd never make it as an actor. My Tripos exempted me from second MB and I made my inquiry of Allen Crockford because, during the weeks I'd carried a spear into corners of Ireland never before penetrated by foreign mercenaries, I'd developed a romantic urge to become an eccentric country GP like Roger Livesey in *A Matter of Life and Death*.

In those days 'grant' was not a word in common usage but I was earning a few bob writing scripts for comedians like Robert 'Bumper Fun Book' Morton and for BBC radio—television was still a minority sport—and Allen Crockford saw no reason why I should give up those jobs while I 'walked the wards'. (He didn't use the phrase but others still did.) In return for his indulgence he extracted an unwritten promise that I would write the St Thomas's Christmas Show which before the war had earned the same sort of reputation as the Footlights Revues.

Allen Crockford was keen to expand the medical school's activities and determined to prevent it from becoming just a place for technical instruction. He had a big say in the selection of students and, though he never tried to emulate the St Mary's policy of buying in rugby players with scholarships, he was always on the look-out for scrum halves, musicians for the hospital orchestra, oarsmen, choristers, editors for the St Thomas gazette, indeed anyone with talent who might occasionally divert other students' attention from their textbooks. He ensured we at least got a chance to develop qualities which today's academic departments are often better at codifying than inculcating. He didn't want St Thomas's students to become a homogeneous group and we ended up heterogeneous almost to a fault. By the time students in my year had qualified, some had played in a team that had won the inter-hospitals rugby, cricket, hockey, or bridge cup, had rowed in a Head of the River crew, or played in an orchestra conducted by the unknown Colin Davis or performed songs written for the Christmas Show by the equally unknown Richard Rodney Bennett.

When I left the Dean's office on the day of my acceptance, I walked through the long Central Corridor which ran parallel with the Thames and linked the ward blocks. It was the High Street of the strange community I'd joined, a bustling place where groups and individuals scurried and strolled, paused and intermingled, regrouped and moved on, gossiping or wrapped in thought: patients smart and patients shabby, nurses with status proclaimed in the colour of their belts or the colour of their uniforms, athletic-looking physiotherapists in white coats with brown belts, midwives in blue serge, lab technicians carrying wire baskets of rubber-bunged test tubes, uniformed porters carrying patients' notes or pushing patients in wheelchairs or patients on trolleys, visitors carrying flowers, patients walking, patients limping, patients swathed in bandages, patients motionless on trolleys wrapped in red blankets and attached by rubber tubes to transfusion bottles, doctors in long white coats, doctors in short white coats, doctors hurrying, doctors standing in groups dangling their stethoscopes behind their backs and deep in earnest conversation, hospital maintenance men and painters carrying buckets and brushes and ladders, kitchen porters pushing closed metal trolleys that gave off a sound of rattling plates and a smell of stew, probationers pushing trolleys laden with steel bowls and drums of sterilized dressings and wooden-cased sphygmomanometers, teaching rounds of consultants and registrars and students on their way to the wards from their assembly point in the Central Hall where the marble busts of their forbears, disguised as laurel-wreathed Greek or Roman nobles, had been swapped around after so many student parties that nobody knew which was which, helmeted policemen looking for the canteen, patients in search of doctors, lady almoners in search of patients, students in search of the nearest exit . . .

The batch of students I joined in my first clinical year ranged in age from early twenties to early thirties because most were ex-servicemen. More than two thirds of us had done our pre-clinical work at Oxbridge; the others had been through the St Thomas's pre-clinical school. There were four women in our year and less than twenty in the medical school. St Thomas's had been one of the last London teaching hospitals to admit women and had capitulated only three years before after resisting change with traditional arguments like not having suitable lavatories.

Some of the ex-service students had led genuinely adventurous lives and won battle decorations. Others liked to titillate those whose experience had been confined to prep and public school. The present professor of general practice in Sheffield, Eric Wilkes, used to claim, for instance, that he'd been a Brigadier in command of a Mobile Bath Unit.

We also had a few students who were labelled 'late vocations'. They included a pharmacist who'd leaped over the counter in middle age and 'Pop' Manley, a retired Indian judge who

was in his sixties and preparing himself to be a medical miss-
ionary. He was so deaf that rumour claimed he didn't pass
his finals until he got a case that didn't require him to hear
anything through a stethoscope. On his first appearance in
the operating theatre, his cap and mask obscured his grey hair
and his facial wrinkles. A pompous young surgeon lectured the
new students on surgical etiquette and hinted how lucky they
were to be apprenticed to genius. When he finished, one of
them stepped forward and said: 'Now, young man, perhaps you
could explain exactly what you're going to try and do.'

We started our clinical careers in Casualty, a word I always
found disturbing because I was used to applying it to a person
not a place. Casualty was a large white tiled hall where the
afflicted sat and waited on benches or in wheelchairs built
like wooden rocking chairs with the rockers replaced with out-
size bicycle wheels. The waiting hall was flanked by smaller
rooms, some with names like Medical Sorting Room, others just
filled with steaming sterilizers and sinks and drainingboards
and shelves that bore enormous bottles of pink carbolic fluid.

In those side rooms, clad in white gowns tied up at the
back, we learned to apply bandages, to lay out trolleys with
rubber sheets and instruments and containers with strange
sounding names like gallipots and porringers, to syringe ears,
swab throats, and give injections of penicillin, the new exciting
drug which worked magic on the carbuncles, boils and septic
fingers our Lambethian patients brought to us in our white
tiled rooms.

Once we could get bandages to stay on fingers (or with
greater difficulty on lower legs) long enough for the patient to
clear the hospital premises, we were promoted to stitching cuts
or even incising abscesses in patients who'd been temporarily
asphyxiated with a mixture of gas and air supplied by one of
our colleagues. For the sake of scientific appearance the gas
supply came from a modern looking machine but the anaesthetic was rarely smooth. Most patients had to be physically
restrained and occasionally instruments and gallipots and even

a student or two flew across the room. Yet when the patients woke they never remembered anything. If we didn't always achieve anaesthesia we never, thank God, failed to induce amnesia.

Casualty was where we first encountered nightingales—the colloquialism for St Thomas's nurses. The Nightingale school, founded by Florence herself, was reputedly the home of an exclusive religious order for the daughters of top drawer families. Even in 1949, we were told, nightingales received direction not to fraternize with medical students. But someone, maybe Hitler, had blown a hole in that tradition and the long hours of the casualty dresser were spiced with mild flirtation; nothing as vulgar as bottom pinching, of course, but lots of significant eye work above the surgical masks and an occasional giggle over the gallipots or the paraffin gauze. Casualty was where we learned one lesson medical students never forget: eyes that enchant above a mask can disenchant at the unmasking. We forged few liaisons in those first few months. Those came later when we visited the wards at night and exchanged sweet nothings over Horlicks in the ward kitchen or occasional sweet somethings in the linen cupboard.

In between our spells in Casualty we attended teaching out-patients. Final year students sat in the front rows, were asked questions and examined patients. We sat in the back row and gawped. The patients we saw were not the serendipitous ebb and flow of hospital out-patients but specimens who'd been specially selected because they had unusual lumps or 'interesting' conditions. I can remember being angered by the arrogance of some of the registrars who bossed the patients about and showed them off as if they were performing animals. And being equally angered by the way patients, if they were old or poor, were patronizingly referred to as Dad or Mum or Pop or Granny without anyone ever asking them if they liked it. But my anger remained unspoken because ours was a docile generation, used to being told what was good for it through seven years of war.

We also attended lectures in which people like Sharpey-Shafer, the professor of medicine, and his reader Tony Dornhorst tried to convince us that clinical medicine was a science and not a collection of old docs' tales. Tony Dornhorst tried to help us understand the circulation with what he called 'an electrical analogy'. His equations, laden with symbols, were more baffling than the hydrodynamics they were supposed to simplify but we could forgive him anything because of the throwaway lines he forced through his stammer. One sleepy summer afternoon he asked a student to name the causes of an enlarged spleen. The student shook himself from half slumber and, playing for time, muttered: 'The causes are legion, sir.'

'Then just give us a co-co-cohort or two,' said Tony Dornhorst.

After Casualty we were attached to medical firms and allotted patients on the wards. It needed a rugged determination and a cultivated insensitivity to question and examine patients who had already endured both processes at the hands of at least six real doctors. The large, airy wards designed by Florence were surprisingly cosy despite their size; they even had a central fireplace where coal glowed in winter and before which most of the great men warmed their behinds while giving us the benefit. We learned to identify some of the noises we were told we should hear through our stethoscopes and became industrious collectors of sputum, urine and gastric wastings. The march of medical science ensured we were also tireless drawers of blood. We chased the veins not with neat and relatively painless syringe needles but with whacking great WR needles. The ward Sisters insisted that the WR needles prevented us from doing unnecessary damage but I always thought them cruel.

Our firm had two consultants, a posse of registrars, a couple of housemen and eight to ten students. Once we had written up our notes on our patients, often copying and rephrasing what the houseman had already written, we had to mug up answers to the questions we guessed might occur to our consultant when we gave the account of our stewardship.

That happened on the weekly teaching round. The consultant stopped at any bed that had his name above it in large letters and asked: 'Whose patient?'

The student responsible then stepped forward and tried to establish the required identity: keen yet humble, bright yet deferential. A few succeeded.

Most of the rounds were amiable affairs. The consultant worked through a repertoire of things he thought we ought to learn, of trick questions, and of carefully-burnished jokes which experience had taught him would last the three months we were under his tutelage. Hector Goadby taught us how to examine patients and how to be kind to them. John Harman and John Anderson tried hard to sharpen our wits, and the endearingly eccentric Evan Jones gave frequent noisy example of just how exciting the diagnosis game could be.

Only one physician played the martinet. There was always tension when Jack Elkington took us round his neurological beds. The student who hadn't done his homework, and occasionally the student who had, was coldly and ruthlessly humiliated before his colleagues. And God help the patient or nurse who made a noise while the great man was talking. One day when we entered the ward, the Elk (inevitable nickname) paused and looked around. Sister had done her work well. Every patient was in bed, neatly lined up with nose the regulation number of inches above the sheet. No bed cover was wrinkled. The nurses stood silently at their posts. No sight nor sound intruded on serenity. The Elk gazed tetchily towards the window.

'The birds are a little noisy this morning, Sister,' he said.

When we played the traditional student game of deciding whom we would want to treat us if we were ill, most settled for a promising young physician who seemed to know his stuff and was nice with it. His name was John Richardson and he was rumoured to have done something clever in the war though we never found out what it was.

Later when we did surgery, obstetrics, and 'others', we extended our acquaintance with the hospital 'characters'—consultants who told good stories or of whom good stories could be told. We also encountered a few less predictable individuals. William Sargant argued with psychotherapeutic passion that psychiatry was merely a matter of applied physiology. Ronnie Furlong taught us orthopaedics in a style that reminded me of Mr Jingle: 'Little Willie . . . climbs tree . . . branch breaks . . . puts out hand . . . green stick. Grandma . . . tiddly after lunch . . . trips over rug . . . dinner fork deformity . . . Colles.'

'Pasty' Barrett, witty and perceptive and with a fine line in professional iconoclasm, was an inveterate practical joker. When a fellow chest surgeon, Sir Clement Price Thomas, received the accolade, 'Pasty' organized a dinner for him and took me along as a putative representative of the Ministry of Health. When the time came for me to propose the Ministerial tribute I announced that there had been a mix up because I came from the Ministry of Agriculture and Fisheries. I then launched into a cabaret performance I used to give of a ministerial public relations man exhorting Britain's trawlermen to improve national kipper productivity. This induced a whole minute of horrified silence before the audience spotted I was sitting next to 'Pasty' and guessed they were the subject of a prank. They then became the most appreciative bunch I've ever known.

Richard Gordon had yet to publish *Doctor in the House* but, when he did, we recognized our world. And he reminded us how great a part hierarchy and anecdote played in our lives and in our assessment of people's worth. We were proud of our 'characters' and retold their tales with pride. Yet our pride was hopelessly blinkered. We never measured our heroes against those alleged to exist elsewhere. I remember 'Pasty' Barrett trying to encourage us to attend lectures at other hospitals but few of us did.

We also had blind spots about parts of our own hospital

which were not on the regular student beat. *Time* magazine took most of us by surprise with a cover picture that revealed St Thomas's had a figure of international repute. Harold Ridley, the ophthalmic surgeon, had been the first man to replace cataract-damaged lenses with acrylic ones. But few of us had noticed because we'd been too busy listening to the 'characters'' stories. Looking back I'm sure we also underestimated the worth of Sharpey-Shafer and people like Geoffrey Bateman whom few recognized as the best surgeon in the hospital because he did ENT in the basement, and Derek Wylie and Harry Churchill Davidson who were busy preparing the textbook that helped establish anaesthesia as a respectable scientific craft.

My children often ask what we looked like in the 'olden days' and I remember exactly each time the BBC reshows an Ealing comedy. Our hair was short and our clothes still wartime utility. Most of us wore grey flannels and tweed jackets, often with leather patches on the elbows. Idiosyncrasy in dress strayed no further than an occasional bow tie or a pair of corduroy trousers. I suspect our accents were pretty uniform too, the cut-glass sort we heard each day on the BBC. Working-class accents were acceptable in patients but not yet on radio or cinema screen where comic underlings were played by cosy souls like Stanley Holloway or Joyce Grenfell using fractured cut-glass voices.

Conformity was a necessary virtue. Eccentricity was tolerated only if it emerged in a gentlemanly form. Active dissent led to a drying up of sources of privilege and patronage. I wonder how much of the conformity was part of a St Thomas's tradition and how much was brought back by ex-service students from their officers' messes. Its observance certainly involved service-like detail. I remember vividly how students who didn't wear a black tie for the full period between King George VI's death and his interment were subjected to unostentatious yet pointed ostracism.

A few clinical students lived at home but most of us lived in digs. St Thomas's House, the students' club across the road from the hospital, had rooms for students on the upper floors but the hospital had taken them over to house foreign workers employed as ward maids and known, because of the colour of their uniforms, as Pinkies. Most student digs were in Chelsea, Battersea, South Kensington or Pimlico. A few intellectuals commuted from Hampstead, exhaling garlic and reading the *New Statesman*, and some lonely souls got stuck in barren single rooms around Earls Court, though most escaped to share flats in less chilly parts of town. Shared flats ranged from well organized households of monastic propriety to notorious establishments in Battersea and Chelsea where the transient population often outnumbered the residents and where the lifestyle was one of dedicated debauchery.

Two sets of digs were highly popular because they were just across the road from the hospital and students living in them could have breakfast and dinner in the nurses' dining-room, though they had to sit at separate tables from the nurses. Number 79 Lambeth Palace Road was the premier digs with clean, well-kept rooms. Number 57, where I managed to insinuate myself after three months, was equally convenient to the hospital but the housekeeping was a furlong or two behind that of 79.

Each room in 57 was lit by gas delivered to the mantles through elaborate brass fittings. Heat came from a gas fire. The supply for both came through a meter which I had to service with shillings, when times were flush, and pennies, when times were harder. The establishment was owned and run by Miss Lang who was old, fat, ponderous and arthritic but essentially well meaning. Every morning she struggled wheezing up the stairs with jugs of hot water, and later, when we were out, with even larger quantities of cold to replenish the jugs that stood in bowls on our marble washstands. She also flicked round the rooms with a feather duster, but as she could neither bend nor stretch she managed to clean only a band of wall that started eighteen inches above the skirting board and ended at shoulder height. Above and below those levels the dust settled undisturbed.

I started in the top floor back and spent six weeks learning to sleep through the sound of the night trains running in and out of Waterloo. After seven months I moved to the second-floor front and spent another six weeks acclimatizing to the noise of the all night trams as they clattered across the points that lay between 57 and the entrance to Casualty across the road. After I'd been there eighteen months, London Transport stopped the trams and I spent another six weeks learning to sleep through the silence.

Like most of the student rooms in Lambeth Palace Road, number 57's second-floor front was alleged to have housed Somerset Maugham when he was a St Thomas's student. It was crammed with Victoriana: a brass fender, a woven table runner that slid off every time I placed anything near it, a dirty lace antimacassar on the back of a springless uneasy chair and a magnificent brass-knobbed bedstead. In winter I used to freeze in that bed because Miss Lang was frugal with her blankets. I piled overcoats on top of me but because I lay on the thinnest mattress I've ever known, and though Miss Lang had packed layers of newspaper between it and the springs, the cold Lambethian fog seeped upwards and caught me *a tergo*. Still it can't have been too bad because I stayed there till I qualified.

A hundred yards along from 57 was St Thomas's House, always called The Club. Housemen, registrars and an occasional consultant might call in at the bar, which had Scotch Ale on draught, but it was really student territory with its club notice-boards, its ground-floor cafeteria where most of us had lunch, its first-floor lounge where we could loiter reading newspapers and magazines and where obsessional bridge players often started to deal at lunch-time and laid down their last hand at one o'clock the following morning, and its ever helpful, ever resourceful head porter, Sid Mullins.

Sid, more than any member of the medical or nursing staff,

was the enduring character in most students' lives. He was a quiet ex-serviceman, lean, dark haired, unostentatious, hard-working and invincibly honest. He showed a remarkable tolerance of the antics indulged in by students at odds with maturity and had a deeply-felt loyalty to the medical school. He would inconvenience himself to unbelievable extents to help any student whom he thought was trying to help the school; he had little time for those who took the school for granted. He was a daily reminder of how simply some people can interpret the complex notion of integrity.

Five or six times a year the Club lounge was transformed into a ballroom when the cricket, rugby or some other sports club held its annual ball. The card tables, chairs, and most of the sofas were carried upstairs and parked in corridors or downstairs and parked in the dining-room. Spectacular quantities of energy and endurance went into decorating the pillared lounge with bunting and balloons, each club trying to outdo all others in the extravagance of its ideas and the effort expended to achieve them.

Come the night of the ball, dinner-jacketed and long-dressed participants rolled in after dinner from Soho restaurants or from parties in digs to dance to the music of such as Sidney Lipton and to quaff Scotch Ale or more exotic drinks served up by amateur barmen under Sid's command. After midnight, the formalities began to melt as the stiff white collars softened in the heat and we locals from 79 or 57 could slip in ticketless to the bar, exchange a pleasantry with Sid, and then wander around the dance floor in search of girls whose partners had inadvertently anaesthetized themselves. After the last waltz most of the lights would go out. Couples with no homes willing to receive them would sit or lie 'snogging' on sofas that had been left strategically against the walls and some amateur would take over the Club piano and tinkle away in half-remembered pastiche of Art Tatum or Carroll Gibbons.

On such a night some tipsy joker slipped me a mickey in the form of a tumbler of gin to which he'd added a dash of orange squash. I was thirsty enough, and had drunk enough, not to notice and I knocked it back in one draught. Soon afterwards the floor started to tilt and jump up and hit me. Luckily Richard Brunel Hawes, known of course as 'Bruno', the occupier of 57's first-floor front, came to my assistance. He wasn't in much better shape than I was but he somehow managed to get me into the lavatory and my head under the cold tap before we set out for home.

I remember us struggling through the fog. I was cold, pale and silent, clutching the railings for support. Bruno was hot, red and noisy, alternating curse with prayer as he tried to drag me along. When we got to 57 he somehow manoeuvred me upstairs and into my room, solicitously got me out of my clothes, into my pyjamas and into bed. I sank into immediate anaesthetized sleep which lasted till I was awakened by angry noises.

Bruno, it seems, had crept quietly from my bedroom and then, overwhelmed by his efforts, had sunk into deep sleep on the landing. The noise that woke me was Miss Lang's reaction to finding him when she arrived with the jugs of hot water.

'Now, now, Mr Hawes,' she said. 'That's hardly being the gentleman, is it? Why can't you behave like nice Mr O'Donnell there, quietly asleep in his bed.'

In December the club lounge became an auditorium fitted with rows of seats that faced the scaffolding stage on which we performed the Christmas Show. It ran for ten nights and two matinees and because few of the audience of some 5,000 would understand private hospital jokes, it contained little incestuous humour.

Between 1949 and 1953 the cast was still, like the Footlights, all male (though we had a female musical director), and the show took the form of self-conscious 'intimate revue' with a lot of lolling about in dinner jackets and musical accompaniment from two pianos, double bass and drums. The humour ranged from desperate attempts at dégagé sophistication to unashamed heartiness and most of it succeeded because we had an indulgent audience.

Thanks to my agreement with Allen Crockford, my involvement with the show was physically demanding. I spent about three months writing it while trying to give the impression I was doing some work in the hospital and making essential cash-earning trips to the BBC Variety Department at Aeolian Hall in Bond Street. We rehearsed nightly for about eight weeks and then the stage crew and I spent a sleepless forty-eight hours in lighting and technical rehearsals. Once we'd opened, we finished off each performance with an all night party for the cast and carefully-selected members of the audience. Then followed a morning's uneasy sleep, a bilious lunch, a listless afternoon, and we were ready to repeat the cycle.

On one night during the run the show was followed by an Old Boys' party at which the stars of yesteryear beguiled us with the turns that had rocked 'em in the aisles in the 'twenties and 'thirties. Most of the music came from Dr Alan Slater whose only professional appointment at the time was that of gliding correspondent to *The Times*. The last night party, which heralded the collapse of our exciting tinsel world, usually ended in oblivion. I remember scaring my mother when, after my first Christmas Show, I arrived home in Yorkshire, went straight to bed and slept continuously for forty-eight hours.

The St Thomas's I knew deserved its reputation as a bastion of conservatism. When I arrived students still spoke with pride of the heroes of '48 who, on the night the NHS was born, painted the embankment opposite the Houses of Parliament with the slogan: 'Boot out Bevan'. I can remember only four students who during the 1950 election acknowledged their allegiance to the Labour Party. And one of those was the son of a Labour MP.

The oft-quoted paradox is that this reactionary institution produces a regular stream of radicals. Definers of the paradox usually quote the pre-war generations that produced the likes of Stephen Taylor, Denis Hill, Richard Doll, Tony Dornhorst and David Cargill. And while St Thomas's can proudly claim to have produced two government Ministers, both of them, Lord Taylor and David Owen, have been members of Labour governments.

The paradox doesn't puzzle those of us who know that in our day there lurked behind the conservative façade as ill-assorted a collection of talents as God, or Allen Crockford, could assemble. We were united only by our loyalty to an institution which, in turn, engendered loyalty to what I hope is still a liberal humanitarian profession.

We didn't allow clinical medicine to dominate our lives and we may not have learned enough medical science to satisfy the enthusiasts. But at least one consultant assured us there would be plenty of time for that after we qualified and, by then, we'd had a chance to learn other things which I don't want to define too closely or people will label them 'vocational training' and start running courses in them. They included a disinclination to take ourselves too seriously and other qualities I deem essential in a civilized society—and oh, how that last phrase reveals my past membership of the Thameside academy.

I didn't know it in 1949 but my notion of a part-time medical student, like that of a part-time doctor or a part-time anything else, was bang in the mainstream of St Thomas's tradition.

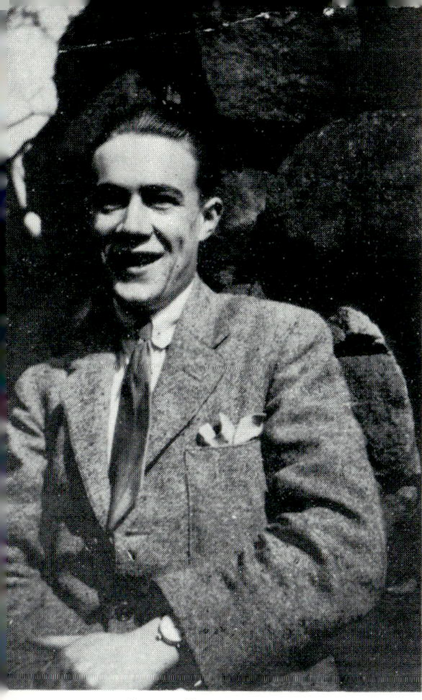

Robert Platt, 1919.

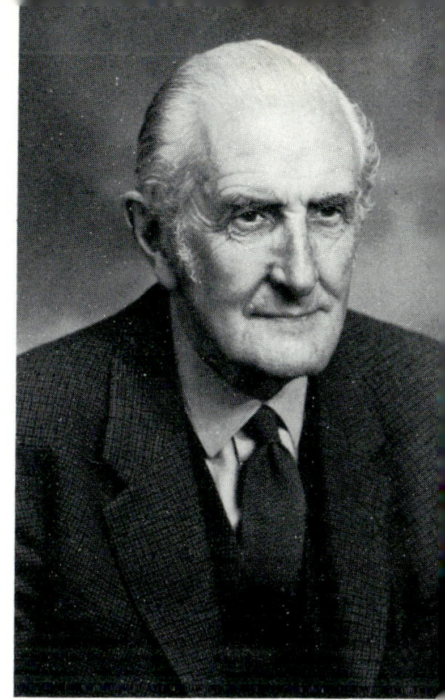

Sir Derrick Dunlop.

William Sargant.

Sheila Sherlock, 1941.

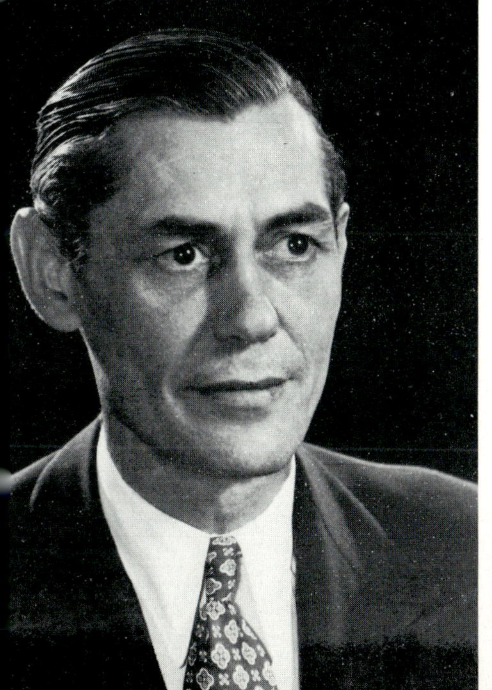

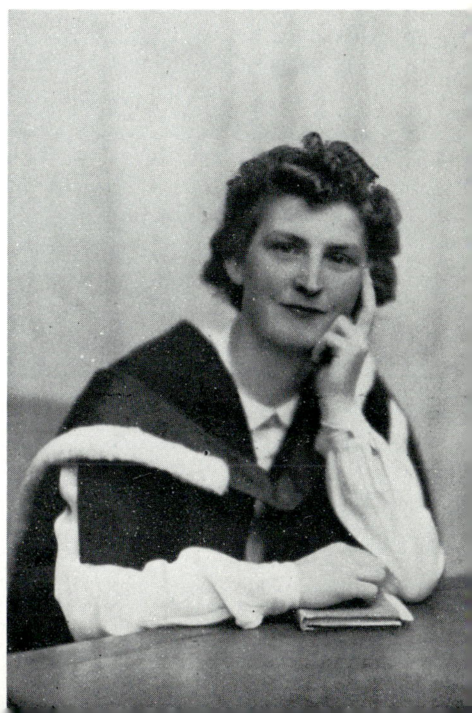

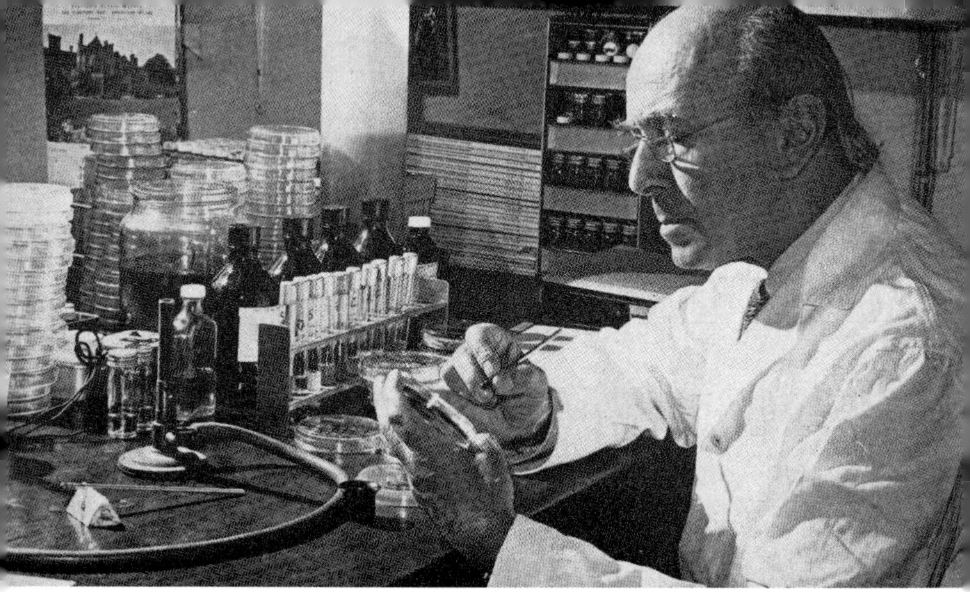

Edward Lowbury.

Ellia Berstock, 1937.

Dannie Abse, 1942.

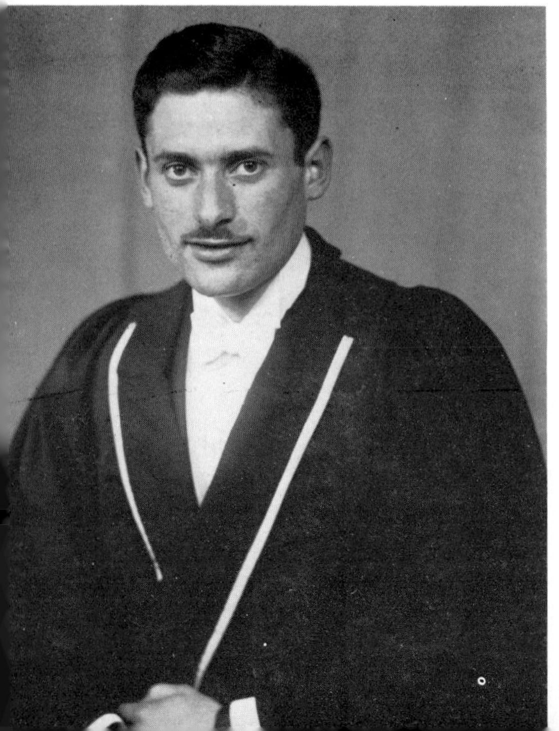

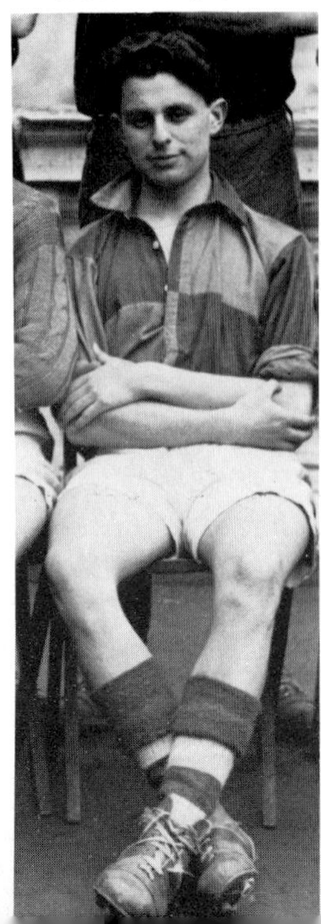

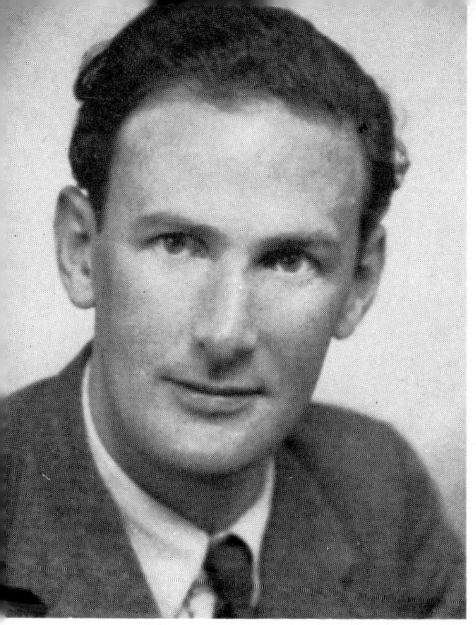

Patrick Trevor-Roper.

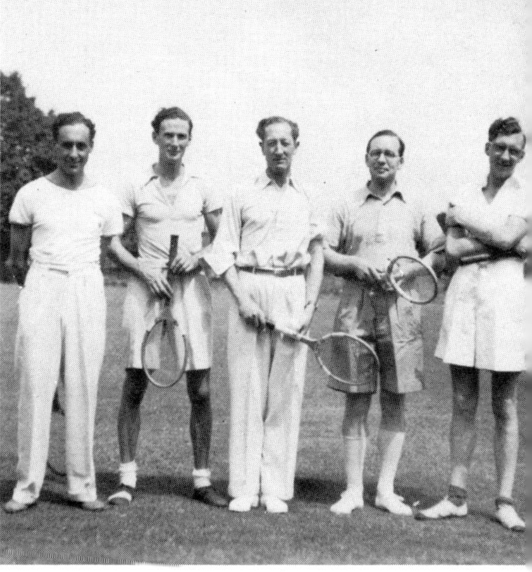

The Westminster Hospital Staff Tennis Team, 1947. Left to right: Frank D'Abreu, Trevor-Roper, Sir Geoffrey Organe, Bryant Evans, Lynn Lockhart-Mummery.

Michael O'Donnell (centre), directing a St Thomas's Christmas show rehearsal.

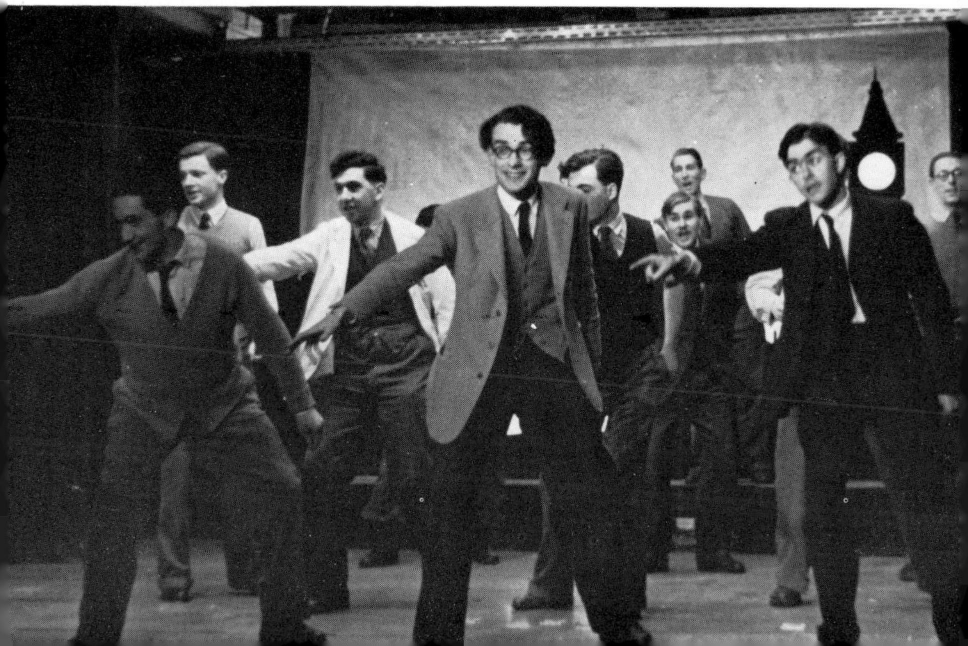

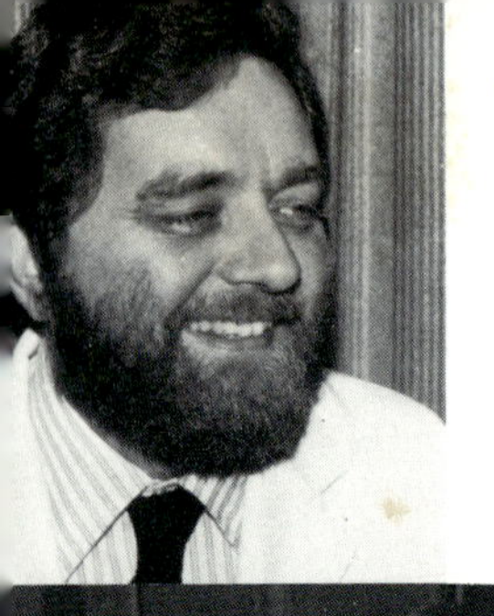

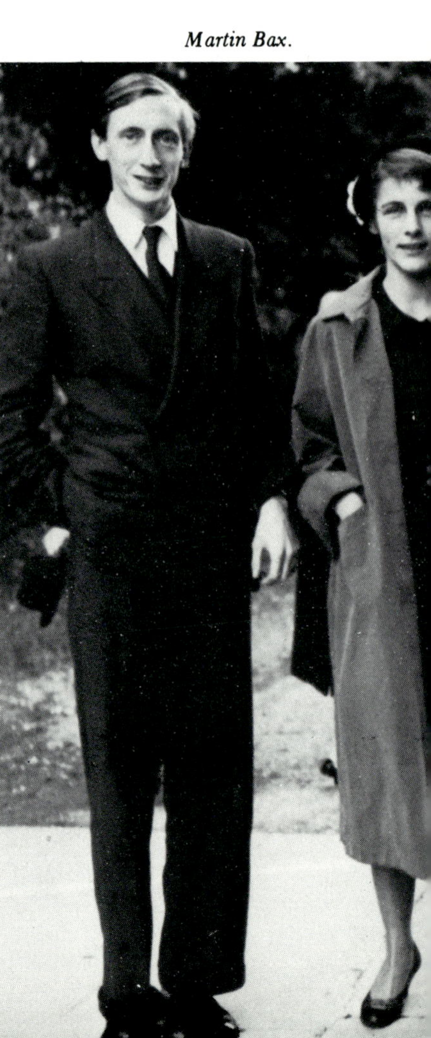

Miriam Stoppard.

Martin Bax.

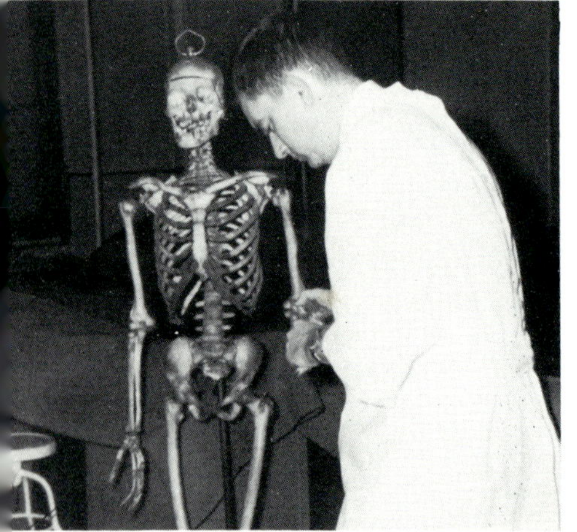

John Stone.

Lesley Isenberg (left).

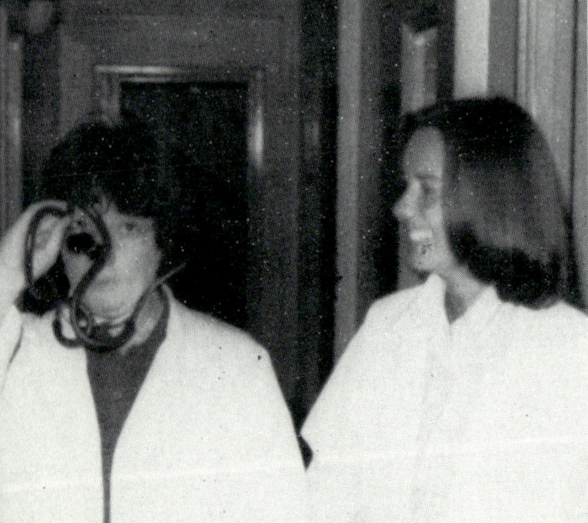

Martin Bax

Martin Bax read Medicine at Oxford University (1952–56) and subsequently did his clinical training at Guy's Hospital. After various house jobs, he joined Spastics International Medical Publications as an editor of their journal Developmental Medicine and Child Neurology. *For several years he ran the Salomon Centre Child Welfare Clinic at Guy's Hospital, and is now research community paediatrician at the Thomas Coram Research Unit of London University. He is Chairman-elect of the Association for Child Psychology and Psychiatry.*

In 1959 he founded the literary magazine Ambit, *which has attracted the work of leading poets and artists. The most recent of his many medical publications is the book* Your Child's First Five Years *(written with Judy Bernal) and his first novel,* The Hospital Ship, *was published in 1976.*

Dr Bax is married with three sons and lives in North London.

I am sitting on the edge of a tall, hard chair. On the edge because I am a small twelve-year-old and if I sat right back in this chair my feet would not quite touch the ground, and I want them on the ground so that I can get up quickly. My parents are in easy chairs, my father is, as usual, silent; my mother is, as usual, not; opposite them across the desk my tall, thin, dreary future headmaster is encouraging my parents to send me to this school. My father has got onto this school in the same way as many people find their doctors —by asking a man from his office with whom he occasionally has a drink in a pub to recommend a good, but less expensive, public school for his son—me. The best thing I shall learn at the school is to like the country it is situated in, and already I have got something of that feeling from the drive across the plain from Salisbury on the way there. Now I am trying to listen to my mother's usual irrelevancies and hoping that the man is not going to speak to me. But he does, or rather he turns to me and makes the following remark: 'Has he thought what he wants to be yet?' I don't have to reply, of course, because my mother jumps in: 'Well, it's early days yet, but he says he wants to be a doctor.'

Before the age of fourteen 50 per cent of future doctors have selected their career. My mother is not directly forcing, but she has ignored the remarks I made when I wished to be an engine driver, milkman, naval officer (a period I can remember well) and latched on to this decision which I suppose I made about becoming a doctor. There seemed no reason to unmake it at twelve, or at any later period in my long student career.

It makes the choices easy. Here I am at fifteen, gone through the first lot of exams where I did best in English Literature, but nevertheless dispatched into the biological Sixth and doing physics, chemistry, zoology and botany. There is a certain pleasure in dabbling with objects, particularly if they are living, and although I spend most of my spare time in the school garden reading Gibbon, I learn about a few things. It is possible to get through the exams if one knows about one place (environment—I choose the sea shore), one flower (I have forgotten which) and one animal (I choose the badger and he stands me in very good stead), but it is none of these that gets me into my first medical school. The bored group of dons who interview me have another thin man at their centre, the Warden. None of them on the interviewing panel are scientists, let alone biologists, and they go over my academic qualifications with a faint air of distaste, and move more surely on to the novels I've been reading. We've been taught about that, and we've all read a statutory Dickens, know about George Eliot and somebody modern, Orwell, probably. The dons are sleepy and suddenly it occurs to me to mention some non-fiction. 'Mr Gibbon,' I say. The thin Warden sits up. 'Gibbon?' he says. 'Yes,' I reply. 'You admire the concise nature of his style?' I don't even have to say yes this time, but simply nod, for he is off, and it is ten minutes before he is at an end, and I am into that medical school even though the rest of the dons are looking even more bored than when we started. They've heard the Warden on Gibbon before.

An anatomy dissecting room. It is half like a classroom, with a dais and a formal master's desk at it. But instead of seats there are plinths with heavily bandaged bodies on them. There are little bits of grey flesh peeking out at the shoulder, at the neck, at the junction of thigh with body, but mostly it is stockinette and mackintosh, and faces like burglars' in stockings which one glances at while this very eminent Professor of Anatomy from Ancient Oxford University makes his introductory remarks to the new students. The remarks are not very memorable and they last only five minutes, when he ends up with the phrase that he is always available for consultation. I never see him again except in his lectures, but he stays on, on this occasion, saying as he finishes his chat: 'I am now going to eat a peach.' A lab technician appears and places a peach, a fruit knife and a plate in front of him, and sure enough, he cuts it neatly into quarters and munches it. It looks juicy and good. We, in fact, are due elsewhere and slip away, leaving him eating.

My dissecting partner and I creep back that afternoon to make an early start. The room is deserted, but we know which body and which arm are ours and we go over with our new dissecting manual (upper limb) and sit down beside the body. The manual vaguely tells you where to start off, but it says nothing about the removal of the 'bandages', which are effectively tied on with string. I try to untie the knots but this is not successful, and finally, taking my brand new dissecting scissors, I cut neatly down over the neck and shoulder, down the upper arm to the elbow. The wrappings fall apart and we peel them off the lower arm in a way which I think resembles (although I had not observed this at that time) the way a woman will take off a stocking. Just as we have completed this two senior students enter the room and march across to the head of our body: 'What on earth are you doing?'

'We're right arm.'

'Have you done bones? You do bones first, you know.'

'Oh.'

'Go into the museum. That's where you do bones.'

So we start to slink off but we are called back.

'Better wrap your arm again or it'll dry out.' But because of my mutiliations we never get the dressings properly on again and the upper arm does indeed dry up before we reach the end of that term. And, when we get to the bones room, all the arm bones are out with wiser students who knew what they ought to be starting with.

Across the road it's physiology. My tutor never excites me and is puzzled as to why I should suggest to him that I might do a different degree from physiology; unhelpful when I ask him much about the scientific basis of human behaviour. His own research for years has been on hot and cold spots: looking for the end organs; I find out that none has ever been demonstrated, and ask him if he has ever found any. 'No,' he says, 'but I keep looking.' 'Where?' I say. 'I take them out of my thigh,' he says. We begin to have to experiment on ourselves, puncture for blood, and one fearful morning swallow a stomach pump and follow it up with a bowl of gruel which we sample back for the next two hours. One student cannot get his stomach tube down and the tutor comes across and tries to force it into him. But there is something wrong with his throat, it won't go down and I wonder what it will be like when one has to do it to a patient.

It is all rather boring really, because I don't allow myself, because none of the other students do, to become excited by the thought of dissecting for five steady terms a dead human body. For some reason, you mustn't get interested in muscle, skin, bone and tissue. It will be more interesting, we say, when we see real patients. I meet my first ones in a holiday job at the local bin. There are five thousand of them, and I am on a chronic ward in the grounds. I am supposed to be a nurse, but in fact we don't do any nursing. We supervise the sweeping of the floor, issue the meals and move the patients at prescribed times from dormitories to day rooms and back again. There is plenty of time to sit in the office and I occupy it by going through the patients' notes. Bill has been there for forty years. His diagnosis is dementia praecox. I haven't found out what that is yet. He is one of our best workers, given his bumper he will polish the floor in a dark place in a passageway all day, and there is always this glassy and slippery patch you have to remember about as you hurry along carrying a tray. In between times Bill stands at the back of the building, furtively looking out for observers, and when he feels he is unwatched moves rapidly round the mat he is standing in front of until he is on the other side of it, and stands there again to wait until he can repeat the manoeuvre. There is something going on in his mind, and he is often a long way away from us, so that when he goes to pee he often comes back unbuttoned with his totally asexual-looking penis hanging out, and when he dresses he forgets buttons, leaves his hair unbrushed and treads down the heels of his shoes. I try (why?) to change some of this, button him up after his trips to the toilet, brush his hair and get his slippers on properly. One morning he comes to me and says, while the charge nurse is standing there: 'Can I have my bumper, sir?' 'Good Lord,' says the charge nurse, 'first time I've heard Bill speak for twenty years.'

Across town I attend dinner to make plans for my wedding. It it to be a somewhat formal affair and I hire myself a morning suit. There are lists of guests being prepared and I am being asked politely who else I would like to come. I hesitate over the fast-fading friendships of school and university and it occurs to me that perhaps I should suggest Bill. I like Bill, but someone has already told me it is wrong to get emotionally involved with one's patients.

There are other wards in the hospital which are locked. Ours is open and the patients can go out, but I have spent a short period on some of the others. Most of the nurses are miners who came down during the slump, because the previous Superintendent thought that music was helpful and hired anybody who could play a brass band instrument. Some of them are kind nurses, some are not. Some hit the patients, some don't. Two years later, when I am doing my own psychiatric appointment, we are waiting for the consultant and discussing the latest newspaper scandal of what goes on in mental hospitals. The young registrar is quite clear about it all. 'Grossly exaggerated. Nobody ever gets hit in a mental hospital.'

There is another student there who has actually been nursing in one for two years in the north country before he decided to read medicine and when he was conscientiously objecting to national service. So we both protest, but it's no use because the registrar knows much more than a medical student, and the other students glance at us askance as he repeats his assertion that violence does not take place, and we don't know what we're talking about. After all, we haven't done any psychiatry yet, have we? We've only just joined this firm.

When you actually reach the hospital—Guy's Hospital with its famous medical school—it is not altogether unpleasing. A broad colonnaded walkway leads you through to a park with tall plane trees and quite pleasant red-brick buildings on either side. The library has ivy-covered walls. Inside, the books are as firmly attached to the walls as the ivy, all behind locked glass doors, and to get one out one has to disturb the librarian, who is secretary of the rugger club and usually on the phone to sporting correspondents of the daily papers.

It is in the colonnade that we make our first contact with a consultant. We, the junior dressers, stand mute while our seniors regale us with anecdotes about the brilliance of the man we are awaiting. About twenty-five yards off stand his registrar and house surgeon. The house surgeon sports a black coat and striped trousers. A short and rather stout man joins them, they chat for a moment or two, and then almost at a run he comes over towards us, scattering us to one side, saying 'Coom on then!' We bounce up the stairs after him to his ward. Later we are, all twenty of us, standing round the bed of a woman whose colon we are to remove the next day—ulcerative colitis. The surgeon uses words to probe her guts, she weeps. He pats her hand and turns to us. 'All these patients are emotional.'

There is little direct contact between the junior dresser and this god, because he teaches the senior students while we listen; we are regaled by his registrar. It is difficult to know how to compete with the sartorial elegance of the house surgeon, particularly given one's somewhat limited funds and wardrobe, but I select a Harris tweed jacket which had been barely worn by an uncle before he died and the restyling of which has led to my first contact with a tailor; this is coupled with my slim-fitting, dark grey, expensive flannels from Hall Bros, in Oxford. But they will not do; one day, as I am crossing the park the black coat of the house surgeon swoops down and he mutters: 'Mr W. does like his students to wear a suit on his rounds.' I never know whether this message emanates from him or from the surgeon.

The patients here are rather different from the chronic sick I'd been nursing a month or two back. The first one is dressed in the most expensive-looking suit and is indeed a businessman from over the river in the City. He comments: 'I'm a guinea-pig, am I?' but he is quite amenable when I frown sternly at him and tell him to take off his clothes, and he climbs meekly onto the couch so that I can probe the lump in his groin. He lies there silently while the registrar questions me about his errant anatomy.

He is not quite the first patient I see, because we have been prepared for this introduction to real patients by an indoctrina-tion course which has taught us the mechanics of examination and exposed us to some chronic patients hired for the occasion (they are actually paid to be examined by these raw students). They must have chronic illnesses to come, of course, but we are nevertheless caught out by the gentle old lady who has had syphilis. The man who runs this course is described as the pre-clinical tutor, but his methods of instruction are formal lectures coupled with questioning of the student, who is expected to provide textbook answers. There is no air of a university in the procedure, and it feels as unintellectual an exercise learning about patients as it did struggling through learning all the names of the knobs on the bones.

If there is an intellectual life which goes with medicine, I am not aware of it at this stage, and seek stimulation elsewhere. My bookish habits are noted. As I am crossing the park one morning I bump into the pre-clinical tutor, still carrying in my hand the book I've been reading on my way into work. His gesture of friendship consists of asking (it is 1956): 'What angry young literature are you reading there, Bax?' I offer him the volume to look at. For some bizarre reason, it is a set of theological essays. It is bewildering to me now to know why I was reading it, but totally bewildering then to the pre-clinical tutor, who hands it back without a word. The lack of intellectual activity is striking among the students, who grind through by fair means or foul; foul I come across in the bio-chemistry exam, when the student opposite me leaves large notes on the sink we share, asking me what on earth he should be doing. Terrified not of corruption, but of the examiner I feebly gesticulate towards bottles he should be mixing, and in exchange he passes me erroneous information about the one part of the practical of which he has some vague comprehension.

Apart from his medicine, the clinical student has, of course, women, sporting matters and cards to occupy his mind. But talk about work, in those moments (and there are many) when we stand around waiting for something to happen, is chiefly anecdote about hospital personalities. The consultants who are caricatured each year in a play are the only heroes of a narrow world. I find them well-informed on their own topics, but seeming to despise even their own colleagues, let alone those in the world outside medicine. They are often arrogant and often rude. It begins to be borne in on me that I shall be very glad to leave this place, and I begin to busy myself with activities outside the medical school.

My fellow students seem to tolerate this and keep telling me anecdotes of their lives. It seems to me that they have an underground life going on which is real and personal to them, while what we observe on the surface and which will become our lives when we are qualified is a pose they are learning to adopt. Late at night the bull-like rugger player begins to tell me about the girls among the nurses who are pregnant, and where they are going to get their abortions. He is worried about one of them and is acquiring some antibiotics to cover her over the course of the procedure. He has just been on holiday to Europe—two nurses and two just-qualified docs in a car. For some extraordinary reason he insured his baggage, and on the way back, reflecting that he would not need the Polaroid dark glasses again, he throws them overboard and claims a fiver from the insurance company.

I don't know how the female medical students fare, but the possibilities of pleasure with members of the opposite sex are excellent for the male medical student because, as I have begun to realize, he is the dominant class in an extremely complex society. Nurses, radiographers, physiotherapists, lab assistants, are all lower down in status and they seem to accept this position and admire not only the fully-qualified species of doctor, but even the fledgling who can preen with success. It is a good world to be in, perhaps.

Late at night we are on surgical emergency and are summoned to see an in-patient, an elderly lady, who has had a surgical procedure but has obstructed again. Her stomach is blown up. We wheel her down to the operating theatre and she lies looking at us. The registrar, who has also been looking anxious, is scrubbing up with a student, and it occurs to me that I ought to be trying to talk to this woman and reassuring her that her life is not in danger, but I can't think of anything to say. A young anaesthetist suddenly pops into the room and says with a warm smile to the patient: 'Hullo! Same again, I'm afraid.' To my surprise, the patient smiles back at him, saying: 'It's you, good.' And I realize that the anaesthetist has in some way got to know this lady and is able to reassure her in a way that I am not. Not that he is anything less than a doctor. As soon as she is on the table he gets a stomach tube into her and finds that the nurse's tube, which is supposed to have aspirated the contents of her stomach, has not been properly in place. He is soon draining off quantities of an evil-looking liquid into a bucket. 'We've struck oil here,' he says. The registrar is, I realize, very uneasy. He has elected to do a second colostomy and keeps saying, 'I hope I've done the right thing, I hope I've done the right thing.' It is difficult to decide whether he is anxious about what the patient will feel in the morning or what the surgeon whose case it is will have to say.

Some things we are taught and some we aren't. On family planning we get one lecture from a man who seems to purvey rubber goods, but an attempt to find out, when we are doing our gynaecology and obstetrics, more about the problem meets with an evasive answer from the consultant, who actually says to me: 'You'll know more about things when you are married yourself.' Which leaves me with the come-back 'Well, I have been married for the last two years, sir.'

A relation of my wife's rings up one morning to tell us that her uncle is in the hospital, and I slide up to the surgical ward to which he has been admitted to try to find out what is happening to him. I find it extremely difficult, even as a student, to get information to answer the questions his relatives are asking, and the consultant is one of those unapproachable ones who doesn't know me, and is not easy to contact. G. lies patiently in the ward not, as it seems to me, getting very much better. I realize that because he had an acute abdominal condition he was admitted to a surgical ward, whereas in fact he ought to be in a medical one. The surgical sister is impatient with him and says he doesn't make much effort. The physician who is called in is able to find out why when he drains a pint and a half of pus from a concealed abscess. In the lunch hour I should go to a clinical lecture every day, but now I find every lunch-time I am sitting by G.'s bed. We talk and he tells me many things but I suppose I miss something by failing to complete my required tally of one hundred clinical lectures. It seems to go on for about a year, he is in and out of hospital, said all the time by the doctors—and after all I am nearly one of them—to be getting better, and visibly looking, alas, worse, and eventually dying.

Soon I can have my chance at these life and death games. In

my final year as a student I command the night emergency service, having the decision allotted to me of calling up my immediate superior, the house surgeon, or actually coping with a patient myself. A drunken Irishman with a black eye comes in. He has a bump, too, on the back of his head, and I have to decide whether he should be admitted for observation. The eye is certainly very swollen, but I keep having to let him go off to the toilet and vomit during the course of examination, and I decide that he can't have been hit very hard. This view of mine is confirmed by his nephew, who comes in supported by two friends to see how his uncle is getting on. It turns out that he is the one who hit him, but before he can say very much about it he passes out on the floor himself and, without asking for any medical assistance, the two friends drag him out. That drunk the nephew can't have hit very hard, I feel, and send the uncle home. He is back two days later with a depressed fracture of the maxilla, and somebody tactfully points out to me that a drunken man can, nevertheless, hit very hard.

The exams keep coming. I discover that there are various different ways of being qualified as a doctor. If I fail my final examination at my ancient university, I could yet practise medicine if I become a Licenciate in Medicine and Surgery of the Society of Apothecaries. It sounds so nice that I go and take their exams, and discover they have a beautiful eighteenth-century hall tucked into the City by Blackfriars Bridge. In the middle of the morning, in the course of a Pathology exam, we are brought a cup of coffee and madeira cake. Afterwards I congratulate one of the Society's porters, who provides us with this civility. 'Ah,' he says, 'before the war we used to give you gentlemen a glass of sherry at the end of the morning.' Ah, I think, it's that olde worlde type of profession I'm joining.

I do fail part of my university final, so with my LMSSA I traipse off to the East End to do my first locum house job. There are open coal fires in the wards and the walls are visibly clean up to only about ten feet. Above that it's work for painters and not for cleaners and, for the moment, they have decided it is safer to leave the germs stuck up there, rather than brush them off on to the patients. I have beds on three wards, so I'm told by the regular house surgeon T., as he shows me hastily round before he goes on holiday, but he gives me no information about what goes on under the different Sisters who have absolute sway on their wards. One is slightly mad, and locks up even the soap when she goes off duty, which makes sterility difficult. The surgeon I am working for likes her as she provides him with a free lunch. I see her carrying the bottles of medicinal Guinness into her office.

After about a week my bleeper buzzes and it's a Sister from a fourth ward. 'Would you come up, one of them's ill.' 'But they're not my patients,' I say. 'Oh yes they are, *Doctor*, didn't T. tell you this is your chronic ward?' I hurry over, apologizing for never having been on her ward. Sister brushes her hair back, says nothing, but leads me to an 86-year-old lady. She has classical pneumonia. The X-ray confirms my physical findings. I treat her and, just as the book says, she recovers from her pneumonia. She stays senile in her bed for a few more years. But Sister is grateful and I pop in every day for a chat. It breaks the day for Sister and her two unqualified helpers, as they struggle with their wardful of chronics.

I am there at last. I don't have an MD, only a bachelorship in Medicine and Chirurgery, in addition to my Master's degree in Arts (all of thirty quid), but somehow this allows me to say I am a doctor. I am just due for a new passport and I have it filled in saying Doctor of Medicine. I collect the degree at a curious ceremony where I have to hold the hand of the Professor of Medicine while some words are recited over me in Latin. To my surprise I am not required to subscribe to the Hippocratic Oath, and indeed it is some years before I even see the text of it. I decide not to apply for a house job at my own teaching hospital, although I am warned by a fatherly man in the employment office that this will have serious consequences for my whole further career. I get a job across town at another medical school.

I begin to ease back from medicine, wondering why I was there in the first place. I am offered a job editing a specialized medical journal. I sit at home correcting manuscripts, but decide I must make a few forays back towards that medical world. I ask to go on a course for adolescent handicapped people. 'Yes,' says the organizer, 'provided it's quite clear that you are not coming as a doctor. These people have had enough of doctors and there's no more you can do for them.' I am saddened to have my hard-earned degree so quickly dismissed, but I acquiesce.

When I arrive at the course I am surprised to find that my name is printed on the list of participants as *Dr* Martin Bax, so my profession is not entirely shrouded. I slip nervously into the common-room and sit down on an uneasy chair. One of the students lurches over to me. He has freckles and red hair and seems rather unsteady on his feet; his voice is a little strange, but he communicates clearly enough.

'Are you really a doctor?' he asks.

'Well, yes, as a matter of fact, I am.'

'Well, you're the first one I've met who's not fat and grumpy.'

A compliment—my first in relation to my new medical status. I determine to unravel the back-hand, and he obligingly elucidates:

'You go into those clinics and there's a big man behind the desk wearing a white coat and he ignores me because he thinks I'm stupid or just a child, and he only talks to my mother. And he doesn't listen to her and we don't get what we want. They wouldn't even sign the form for me to have a tricycle.'

They—the doctors—yes, I think, and I've always wanted to be one.

Miriam Stoppard

Miriam Stoppard (née Stern, formerly Moore-Robinson) was born in 1937. She was educated at Newcastle Central High School before studying medicine at the Royal Free Hospital, London, and at King's College Medical School, University of Durham. After qualifying in 1961 she gained her MRCP (University of London) in 1964 and her MD (University of Newcastle) in 1966. From 1966–68 she was Senior Registrar in Dermatology at the University of Bristol.

In 1968 she joined Syntex Pharmaceuticals Ltd, and in April 1977 became its Managing Director. She has contributed many papers to the medical journals, and is a frequent broadcaster on radio and television. She is married to the dramatist Tom Stoppard and has two sons and two stepsons.

I was a failed Girton entrant with no medical connections. Stifling the unjust suspicion that these two states of being might not be unrelated, I arrived in the end—by which I mean at the age of eighteen—at the Royal Free, London, for three years of pre-clinical studies. That was followed by clinical studies at King's College, Newcastle-on-Tyne, my home town, but by that time as a woman of the world (Newcastle and London) I had grown up, so in my reminiscent moods I tend to dwell more on the Royal Free, where for the first time in my life I opened my eyes and looked around.

However, it was in Girton—if not *at* Girton—that my medical education, in a broad sense, properly began. Would-be Cambridge medical students spend a week in the college of their choice—Girton or Newnham for female would-be's in 1954—sitting various examinations, written, practical, oral and, as I found out, social.

I arrived dressed to what passed at Newcastle Central High for the nines, which in my case included neat black suede shoes with Louis heels, the height of fashion and the most treasured shoes I had ever possessed. I found almost everybody else wearing brown flat shoes, dark green skirts, cream blouses and school ties. It would be nice to report that I made them feel thoroughly upstaged, but with numbers on their side their disapproval came easily. I shrank. And how was it that the school-tie brigade knew their way around so confidently, exercising territorial rights and grandly snubbing outsiders?

I learned that they were hard cases from Cheltenham Ladies' College, some of them up for the third time. Heavens. School ties, perhaps, but their savoir faire was stunning. I was an amateur among professionals. My rivals for one of the six Girton places left me standing at the gates.

This was made plainest to me at the group interview which customarily takes place during the examinations week. After dinner one evening, four of us meekly entered the tutor's study at the appointed hour. It turned out, however, that I was the only one whose meekness was the real thing.

My one memory of that awful experience is being asked which particular branch of medicine we intended to specialize in after we graduated. My God, we weren't even students yet. The first young lady said she hoped to join her uncle at an African university to take up a career in tropical medicine. The second young lady felt she would like to follow her mother into anaesthetics. The third young lady had talked things over with her physician father and had a yen to take advantage of his connections with Great Ormond Street and become a paediatrician.

As my turn approached I realized that I had seriously missed out on fireside chats with medically-qualified relatives. I had been set on a medical course at the age of six as the elder daughter of a tailor who was determined that his first-born, regardless of gender, would be a doctor. At high school I had been streamed into science as soon as my teachers learned of this, and, as though on automatic pilot, I found myself in the Science Sixth trying for exemption from first MB.

And now here I was at Cambridge—no, *in* Cambridge— being asked what I intended to *specialize* in before I had begun to get even a *general* idea of medicine. I said as much, and the letter turning me down arrived about ten days later. It took me weeks to get over the regret that I would never be punted about under the willows by elegant young men in pale blue.

Worse still, while I knew that there was unlikely to be much punting by elegant young men at the Royal Free, I didn't realize just how unlikely it was. No one had told me that the Royal Free was for women—founded by women, run by women and attended by women. It had been so since 1874—when it was established to enable women to qualify as doctors for the first time—and it was only the advent of the National Health Service that brought about a change of its charter to admit a ten per cent intake of men.

It didn't occur to me at the time that the feminist history of my medical school was something to take pride in. Back in 1858 when the first medical register was drawn up there was only one woman on it, Dr Elizabeth Blackwell, and she was there more or less by accident, having qualified in America. The ranks closed again for a mere seven years before another of these damned females got in—Elizabeth Garrett Anderson, who had with great determination won her membership of the London Society of Apothecaries.

This unseemly rush of women caused the Society to alter its rules to exclude women from its examinations, and effectively disbarred women from studying medicine in London. Up in Edinburgh at about this time, Miss Sophia Jex-Blake and four colleagues were fighting the university to enable women to enter the medical school there. They failed, and as a result money was raised in London to buy the lease of a house in Henrietta Street, Covent Garden. It was here that the first medical school for women opened its doors in October 1874, with 14 pre-clinical students.

Three years later—exactly a century ago as I write—the Royal Free Hospital admitted the first women students to its wards for clinical instruction, and it only took a couple of decades for this relationship to be formalized in the new name of what became the London (Royal Free Hospital) School of Medicine for Women.

Had I known any of this at the time I wouldn't have been quite so horrified when I timidly opened the door of the most beautiful common-room in London and found it filled to bursting with chattering girls. Not a man in sight, elegant or otherwise. No, there was one man—a fifth-year student who made a habit of coming in on the first day of the academic year to cast his eye over the new intake. It's not that I was man-mad, but after seven years in a girls' school I thought I had flown the nest, and here I was, apparently back in another one. I looked round the room. Six more years of this. What had I done? I wanted to catch the first train home.

On the other hand, there was London. My bit of Tyneside was short on reliable references to the essential London. I carried around with me images of pearly kings and queens, beefeaters, and a knees-up at the Old Bull and Bush, and these images accompanied me in the Flying Scot, and then down into the Underground. It was dusk when I surfaced to the pavement, fresh from the satanic North. I couldn't believe my eyes. Oh, the sophistication of it all! And how cosmopolitan! Those exotic shops, those grand buildings, luminescent coffee bars and chic restaurants. Everyone seemed to be dressed in a way that would have turned heads where I had come from. The weight of my suitcase compelled me to stop every ten yards or so, but I didn't mind that. I gazed and gazed. So this was London! The hub of the Empire, the seething centre of the Big Apple. Actually, I had got out at Hampstead, and this was not so much London as Heath Street, NW3. But no supporting act ever got a better audience. It was love at first sight.

When I got around to discovering the main feature, it turned out to fulfil every promise, an endlessly thrilling treasure house, a rock candy mountain where, even if the fountains didn't quite run lemonade, theatres were often 'papered' with free or half-price seats for medical students, and retrospective exhibitions of Kandinsky, Kokoschka and Klee turned up within one term, where coffee with froth on top had just been invented and spaghetti bolognese just discovered. Lyons Corner House was still offering all you could eat for 7s 6d, and Chris Barber was still filling his Oxford

Street club so tight that there was no room to jive and it was life enough to stand there and let the Dixieland hit you.

When was all this? To name a date doesn't convey the period. But one night at the jazz club, when the band was about to take a break, Chris Barber announced that some of his musicians had formed a sort of group who would play in the intermission. The music had an unfamiliar twang which most of us dismissed out of hand. Some time later when that Lonnie Donegan sound had spread like Spanish 'flu, I realized that I had witnessed the birth of skiffle. *That's* when it was. And if they're still doing 'The Good Old Days' on TV in 2001, as far as I'm concerned it'll be someone singing 'Big Butter and Egg Man' to an audience wearing corduroy suits and sack dresses.

In short, I was soon glad I hadn't caught the train home. There were seventy-eight of us women in my year, tempered, if that's the word, by six men. The proportion never seemed that bad because we also had among us ten students from the Royal Dental Hospital who joined us to do basic pre-clinical studies. They seemed to me to have a certain raffishness and lack of seriousness which greatly lightened our lives. It was one of these young men who on looking round the common-room one morning during coffee-break remarked, 'Yes, the women here have everything a man could wish for—moustaches, broad shoulders, big muscles . . .'

As for the medicine, I was quite overawed by it. Getting a place at medical school was, despite all my conditioning, or because of it, more than I had even dreamed of. Being allowed to walk the corridors, to work in the labs, sit in the lecture theatres, these were privileges I felt I would never live up to.

During the first few weeks it was the local jargon, the professional language of medicine, which seemed to be the key to acceptance for others, and the barrier to acceptance for me. I was in new country and, as for all strangers, it was the language which defined those who belonged and those who (so far) did not. During my first term I once strayed into a seminar for clinical students. The registrar was asking a question about the treatment of a patient with paralytic ileus. 'Gastric suction and the institution of intravenous infusions,' replied one of the group. *Oh heavens*, I thought in panic, *how will I ever learn it?*—little knowing that three years later I would have not only learned it but sometimes discarded it, so that the phrase I had overheard that day would come out as 'drip and suck'.

More formal medical language, however, had its uses, and not always to impress. One of my lecturers at the Royal Free who had the duty of saying grace before dinner frequently couldn't come up with the proper Latin. While we bowed our heads, he would mutter: 'Levator labii superioris alaeque nasi', which was the name of a small muscle running down the side of the nose to the upper lip.

Anatomy and physiology were taught in the traditional manner at the Royal Free, and as in most other medical schools with their roots in the nineteenth century, the focus of the anatomy department was a long room commonly referred to as the Long Room. In our case, this was a high-ceilinged, marble-floored room running the whole length of the top floor, and lit from above by large skylights. The two sides were lined with metal tables. We worked in groups of four round our cadaver, which over the period of the anatomy course rather endeared itself to us as we delved systematically into its organs. We took turns at dissection, one of each pair working on the body while the other read out instructions from the dissection manual.

As we were assigned to right or left, we became familiar with one-sided anatomy, and much less familiar with the mirror image. Consequently, years later in the operating theatre I was still making mental adjustments when the surgery was going on on the 'wrong' side of the patient.

Our Long Room impedimenta was considerable and included dissection kits, numerous reference books, anatomical maps and atlases. Being fastidious, I preferred the atlas to the real thing, and in fact that book of beautifully-drawn and coloured plates became one of my most prized possessions. I was utterly content as I pored tirelessly over those pages, and not quite so carried away when following up the dissections in the raw.

But the main memory is the smell. The smell of formalin pervaded the whole upper floor of the building, and from the very first morning there it stuck to our hands, hair and clothes. We all quickly learned to reserve one dress to wear for dissection, and even so my wardrobe stank like a morgue when I opened the door.

But the smell I could cope with. Vivas were never less than terrifying. Right to the end I never learned how to take them calmly. We had a viva every Friday on the week's dissection, and were examined by the tutors in turn. The Professor was a reticent and stoical woman respected by all of us, not least because we never saw her without an orthopaedic collar which she wore for a mysterious neck complaint.

I had dreadful cause to remember being tested by her on the bones of the pelvic girdle. She handed me a bone.

'Point out the anterior superior iliac spine.'

Ho hum.

'Well, feel your own, if you can't find it on the specimen.'

Er.

'Come along, young lady, everyone has an anterior superior iliac spine. Feel yours.'

I prod at my hip.

'Here, you'd better let me . . .'

She prods at my hip. She keeps prodding.

'Oh, I see. Oh dear.'

From then on I was the Girl Too Fat To Feel Her Anterior Superior Iliac Spine.

But others had, if anything, even less flattering handles, like the Girl Who Bought Her Clothes From The Wrong End of Oxford Street. Most of us were almost as interested in clothes as in medicine (the rest of us were even more interested in clothes than in medicine). Each new outfit was dissected as minutely in the common-room as the cadavers were in the Long Room, a matter of constant interest and speculation. Girls passed into local history for achievements as far removed from medicine as being the first into pointed toes and stiletto heels, or wearing so many frothy petticoats that on leaning over the chemistry bench the flash of thigh stopped lecturers in their tracks.

After spending seven years mostly in chocolate brown, I was bowled over by the freedom to attend classes in mufti. This was the time when the word 'boutique' was turning from a foreign word into an English one, and the heart of boutique-land was just close enough to enable me to make it to a shoe-shop in the lunch hour and be back in time for biochemistry.

In lunch hours when I wasn't chasing into the West End for bargains, I could saunter the quarter mile to the brand new University of London Union. I explored it with a fierce sense of possessiveness. I swam in *my* university swimming pool, ate in *my* university cafeteria, I read in *my* Quiet Room, I studied in *my* Library, I played ping-pong in *my* table tennis room, I glanced at newspapers in *my* lounge, I met friends in *my* bar. Best of all through ULU I overcame the isolation of being a member of a medical school as opposed to a college. (When the newness of our medical school wore off we envied the luckier ones who were studying medicine alongside several other disciplines; those at King's College Hospital and University College Hospital, the latter having all faculties except Divinity, 'The Godless Towers of Gower Street'). At ULU we gladly found ourselves exposed to historians, engineers and linguists.

But I mustn't belittle what was a genuinely thrilling interest in the real business of the day, and in fact it was biochemistry which for me became and remained the most thrilling of subjects. The exploration into the very metabolism of cells, the building blocks of the body, is still the ultimate wonder. However, I remember my first biochemistry lecture for a less sober reason. The lecturer, who seemed a serious and shy sort of chap, introduced us to some of the wealth of data that lay waiting in a specimen of urine for the persistent investigator. He held up a test-tube of liquid that shone golden in the lights of the lecture theatre.

'You can learn a great deal about what's going on in the body,' he said, 'by getting a urine sample and doing a very simple test. Taste it.'

With fascinated horror we watched him dip a finger into the test-tube, remove it, and suck with relish.

'May I call upon you for a volunteer to corroborate what I say.'

There wasn't a movement in the class.

'Oh, come along. You will soon learn that to practise well, a little courage is needed.'

No one moved.

He pointed to a man in the first row.

'You come and try.'

As the unfortunate fellow stumbled to the front of the class, our ninety hearts went with him. He dipped his finger into the urine and forced it into his mouth.

'Ladies and gentlemen,' said the lecturer, 'here we have an example of the first rule in medicine. *The importance of observation.* Our colleague dipped his forefinger into the test-tube and with understandable reluctance tasted it. Had he observed me closely he would have seen that although I dipped in my forefinger, I put my middle finger into my mouth.'

Not all lessons stuck as well as the importance of observation, but one way or another we learned that there was more to medicine than just medicine. Much later I had to re-learn the lesson that one should always hear a patient out. This was when I was doing my stint in the hospital clinical chemistry laboratory. Wednesday was sperm-count day, and each patient was welcomed with a bottle and a card and directed to a cubicle where he could produce a sample. I recognized that sheepish look on a patient one Wednesday morning, gave him his bottle and his card, and firmly directed him, with instructions, into the loo. He emerged triumphant but bewildered. As he handed me his bottle, he said, 'I wasn't told about anything like this. The doctor said I should come to see you because he thought I was a bit anaemic.'

It is a curious fact (though, of course, on second thoughts it is not curious at all) that most people's repertoire of medical anecdotes concerns in one way or another the reproductive and excretory organs. In my combined experience as medical student and doctor, the incident which became joyfully and endlessly retold, occurred when on the Grand Ward Round one of our Senior Consultants was on his knees in the classical manner by a patient's bed, the better to make his extremely intimate exploration. In the middle of it, he looked up, his finger still plunged into one of the body's recesses, and gasped. 'Oh, Sister,' he said with infinite reproach. We all looked at one another in horror. Had we missed something?

'Oh, Sister,' he repeated, groaning aloud. 'I have seen the new moon through glass.'

We turned our money over and moved to the next bed.

While we were studying for second MB (the examination which ended the pre-clinical course and, if passed, would open the door for me to the hospital wards in Newcastle), I turned a corner. First, I discovered in myself the ability to come to grips with the discipline needed for long unbroken periods of study; in fact, I'd discovered the pleasure of 'the Stacks', that part of the library where the oldest texts are stacked into small cubicles, each furnished with a desk and chair.

Here, by some tacit agreement, any student who established herself or himself in the stacks could secure the right of occupancy by leaving papers and books on the desk. I could go away for hours, even days, but the territory was inviolable, and I could return certain that not even a piece of paper would have been disturbed. I'd creep into my stack, silently acknowledging the other regulars, and there I was, a thrilled and grateful member of the fraternity.

The other discovery was more important. From about three months before the second MB, the class split up into groups of five or six to study and revise. From among the class I lit on a chap called Mike and his girlfriend Margaret, who shared a table with me in anatomy class. They seemed bright, lively and thorough. I felt that if I could keep up with Mike I'd do all right. What I didn't quite know was that Mike had the best brain in the class. With some luck and some judgment, I had picked a pacemaker. He taught me to work from basic principles, and to trust to memory as little as possible. But above all he showed me relationships between seemingly unconnected pieces of information, revealing a grand design to the pre-clinical sciences which had escaped me. He reduced a mass of material to a form that was simple, general, memorable and, most of all, exciting to me. 'A renal glomerulus is a modified sweat gland,' Mike would say, and suddenly I would understand. *Of course, of course!* It seemed to me then, at last, that I might indeed make a doctor.

Returning to my hometown to continue my studies at King's College, Newcastle, was like taking an ice-cold shower. For one thing the College was multidisciplinary, all the disciplines sharing the campus so one jostled with engineers, historians and linguists in the 'Bun Room'. For another the College was situated in the centre of the city and was an integral part of it spiritually as well as physically. Tynesiders were proud of their College, interested in it and the people who went there. The feeling was tangible, no more the metropolitan anonymity. More important, the Royal Victoria Infirmary where we were to train drained a huge catchment area, the whole of the northern triangle of England, so there was no shortage of clinical material and to my delight I found that seven or eight patients on a ward were allocated to each student; in London sometimes the reverse was true. And that was not the only ratio which was reversed—men outnumbered women by ten to one.

Newcastle was a good place to be studying medicine in 1958.

We found ourselves in the thick of the controversy about medical education; pure or applied? by subject or by system? written examination by essay or multiple-choice questions? Through the offices of George Smart, our Professor of Medicine and a person eager to make the teaching of medicine more efficient, we found ourselves trying out new methods of being taught or being examined, each step a step forward, most nonetheless pretty scary. We were the first medical students who completed a multiple-choice question paper as part of the MB examination—an innovation quickly adopted and legitimized by the Royal College of Physicians largely due to the data we furnished to George Smart.

Our Professor of Medicine attracted excellence and creativity like moths to a flame. One of his brightest protégés was Reg Hall who was honoured with a personal chair within an almost unseemly short time of qualifying. I remember him in the old days when as a newly appointed house-officer he was given the unheard of and dubious honour of teaching the junior clinical students of whom I was one. One morning when Reg was in full flood on the cardiac complications of thyrotoxicosis Professor Smart came on to the ward with a visiting physician and they stopped for a few moments to listen to Reg. As they moved on the visitor turned to Smart and conjectured:

'That your Senior Registrar, then?'

'Good heavens no, he's my houseman,' rejoined Smart.

'Phew,' said the visitor pensively, 'I'm lucky if my houseman can tell me the heart goes lub-dub.'

Whilst general medicine was my first love from the start, most of the excitement was in surgery and it was George Feggetter who provided it. I was the first woman to work on his unit in thirteen years and all the staff shared my nervousness, including Mr Feggetter. Notwithstanding, I was thrown straight into the deep end (absolutely hair-raising but I became a doctor virtually overnight) and was expected to pull my weight in every aspect of the unit's work. After a particularly difficult and strenuous night on 'reception' for emergency surgical cases I faced him at 8.30 am, pale and badly in need of sleep. He wanted to know how the patients who had been operated on during the night were progressing. He fingered his moustache as he looked down at the overnight nursing records.

'Miss Stern [as I then was], what's this man's haemoglobin?'

'Sir, I've only just come on to the ward. I haven't checked it yet.'

'Do you know, Miss Stern, when I was in the desert campaign [he had been a brigadier] it was not uncommon to receive 3000 wounded in one night. And in the morning when I asked my adjutant for their haemoglobins, he knew every one.'

It was just as well he kept me up to scratch because I had to serve two months of my surgical tenure on the Orthopaedic Unit. Again I was breaking new ground. The orthopods shunned women and I was the first in a long time. The reason for their reluctance became obvious the first time I was faced with a fractured femur. The prospect of having to treat a fractured femur paralysed me with fear. However would I manage the splint? The Steiman's pin? Would I be taken in by the patient's classically good condition and undertransfuse? As the time drew near for my orthopaedic stint I became sleepless with worry. But there was no way I could escape a fractured femur in two months. He arrived in the first week. Everything went well until I came to the Steiman's pin. I struggled, pushed, heaved but could make no headway. The anaesthetist began to complain, this was a two-minute job and I was taking much too long. I asked him to relax the patient more.

'He is relaxed,' came the reply. Finally I had to admit I just wasn't strong enough to push the pin through the tibial tubercle.

'Here, use this.' He handed me the wooden mallet from his trolley which was used to knock open the valves on the gas cylinders. The pin went through like a dream. The story went round the Anaesthetic Department in a flash. From then on whenever an anaesthetist was called to help me with a fractured femur, and I had plenty, he came swinging a wooden mallet.

In a teaching hospital the serious business of treating patients vies with the serious business of taking post-graduate examinations. It was especially important then, and probably still is, for a woman to win her spurs. The most effective way of doing this was to gain the MRCP or FRCS qualifications. Being more attracted to medicine I was tilting at the Royal College of Physicians. We would-be MRCP candidates talked, ate, drank and slept the 'membership'. On the first occasion however it was of no avail. My sense of failure was such that I was hardly comforted by the kind words of David Kerr, who, on meeting me the morning following the bad news, said, 'Never mind, Miriam, none of us would have talked to you if you'd got it first time.' The post-mortems on where I'd gone wrong were endless. One of my much-envied friends who'd passed the exam offered philosophically, 'There's no advice I can give you, the day that you're going to pass, all your cards will stand up. It's as simple as that.'

I had good reason to remember his observation when preparing for another shot at the Holy Grail of medicine. The night before I was leaving for London I asked a radiologist if he would take me through a few X-rays, as it was quite common for the examiner to slot an X-ray into the viewing box and ask the candidate to comment. We spent an hour discussing the classical pictures that came up regularly. Just as we were packing up he said, 'I dug this out for you. That old hoary one —reticular mottling of the lung.' Fine, I thought, I know all about this. It turned out to be a real rarity—Histoplasmosis— a fungus disease commonest in certain areas of the United States. In a couple of minutes he outlined the distinguishing features of the disease down to the fine differences in the shadows of Histoplasmosis and Cystocercosis . . . more elongated . . . denser at one end, etc.

The following morning after an ECG and an electrophoretic strip the examiner reached for an X-ray and held it up in front of the illuminated box. Histoplasmosis! I couldn't believe my eyes. Control yourself, girl, give the information sensibly and slowly. So I embarked on a list of the commoner causes of mottling of the lungs.

'Well now, young lady, if your patient had just returned from a trip to India what would you think of?'

'Cystocercosis—but it isn't.'

'Oh and why?'

'More elongated, denser at one end . . .'

'Do you think you know what this is?'

'Yes, sir.'

'What is it then?'

'Histoplasmosis.'

'Oh really? And what is histoplasmosis?'

'A fungus disease common in certain parts of . . .'

Yes, the day you pass your cards just stand up.

The most enjoyable memories however, are not the savouring of small triumphs but the recollection of humorous incidents; our first day as junior students in a Gynaecology Clinic for instance, each of us praying we won't be the one asked to do an internal examination. The moment comes.

'You there, examine that patient in Cubicle Two.' In goes one of the most intrepid of our number. He emerges quite a while later.

'Well, what did you find?' As he describes the detailed findings of his researches it becomes obvious that he has indeed performed an internal examination.

'You fool,' explodes the registrar. 'Didn't you realize the girl was a virgin? What will her boyfriend say?'

'Oh don't worry, sir, I'll give her a note for him saying I did it.'

John Stone

John Stone was born in Jackson, Mississippi, in 1936. He received his MD degree from Washington University in St Louis (Missouri) in 1962, and subsequently trained for two years at the University of Rochester, New York. He completed his training in Internal Medicine and Cardiology at Emory University School of Medicine in Atlanta, Georgia. He is now Professor of Medicine (Cardiology), Director of the Division of General Medicine, and Director of the Emergency Medicine Residency at Grady Memorial Hospital/Emory University School of Medicine.

Dr Stone is the author of several medical papers relating to his specialty and is Associate Editor of Principles and Practice of Emergency Medicine *(W. B. Saunders, 1978). He has also published a book of poetry,* The Smell of Matches *(1972).*

Such things often begin with a flight of stairs. Or so it seems to me. The stairs I mean are those which led from the first floor of the basic science building at Washington University School of Medicine in St Louis, Missouri, up to the floors above with all their unknowns and strange instruments, and unique smells, and people in white coats deep in their various work.

Actually, of course, medical school begins with getting into medical school. And a lot of people want to get in. Exactly when I decided I wanted to be a physician, I don't remember. There were precedents in my family: my grandfather and an uncle were physicians. I do know that I had decided at least ten years before I walked up that flight of stairs for the first time. In fact I don't recall ever considering seriously anything other than medicine. I went to college in the capital city of Mississippi—Jackson—to a small Methodist-related college called Millsaps College, where I majored in Chemistry, as most pre-medical students did. Each fall or winter, representatives from several medical schools toured the South, talking with prospective students, especially those who seemed promising in terms of their scholastic record. The representative from Washington University always interviewed in the Chemistry Department of my college. In both my sophomore and junior years, I went by while he was there, hoping to simply put my name in the hat, even though it was clearly premature to do so. Both times, the interviewer, the Registrar, was pleasant enough, but simply waved me away telling me to come back next year. In my senior year, there was a different interviewer there, a tall pleasant man, a neuroanatomist with whom I had a nice chat. I knew that I had a good scholastic record, and he had my entire record before him. At the end of the interview, in as undramatic a fashion as one could expect, he simply said, 'We'd like for you to come to Washington University and we're prepared to offer you a scholarship.' The days of decision-making as to where to go to medical school were then over.

But to go back a bit: in the junior year of college, it was required that pre-medical students take a test of aptitude, which I took and found both pleasurable, as tests go, and frustrating. The only part of the test that was really frustrating was that portion devoted to 'spatial' arrangements of geometric figures: one figure on the left of the page was to be compared with four figures on the right of the page and I was asked to choose which of the four on the right could be turned over or rotated to become the same as the one on the left. If my description of the task is difficult to convey, the task itself seemed, in short, ridiculous. The remainder of the test was almost fun; the spatial part I simply chose not to complete. Several weeks later, after the test results had been returned to the Dean of Men, I was called into his office for a discussion of my future plans. You must remember that I was at that time a junior student, with almost three years of college behind me and a firm commitment toward science and pre-medical studies. The occasion of my discussion with the Dean of Men was therefore of great interest to me. He began explaining the test results to me in a very positive way. He stated, for example, that I had done extremely well on the word-aptitude or language-aptitude portion of the test, scoring in a high percentile. Then, looking down the column of figures, he said, 'You didn't do well at all on the spatial portion of the test.' I explained to him that I had simply found it boring. He pointed out, in his best academic tone, 'But I understand that you want to be a doctor. And you didn't do well on the spatial portion of this test. What if, let's imagine, you become a doctor and you're operating and *you can't find the appendix*?' It was, of course, absolute nonsense, but one of the more nearly perfect examples of inappropriate extrapolation of test results. I persevered toward medical school in spite of his parting suggestion to me that I'd do well, based on the test results, as an English teacher. (I like to think I probably would have! But that's another story.)

The scholarship which had been offered by Washington University was absolutely vital. Otherwise, I might not have gone. My father died of a heart attack while I was a senior in high school; although the family was protected by insurance, my younger brother and sister remained to be educated after me and the scholarship was a decisive factor in where to enter medical school.

St Louis was to be the big city for me. Jackson, Mississippi, was the capital of the State, but nevertheless was a town of about 100,000, still quite small in relative terms. After finishing college in June, 1958, I married a woman whom I had known since high school and who shared my aspirations for the future, having herself obtained a degree in Elementary Education and Music at a nearby women's college. We then set off in a quite-used brown 1951 Dodge on the 500-mile trip to St Louis.

At the end of that trip, there were, in fact, two flights of stairs. One flight, at the School of Medicine, led up to Anatomy and Physiology and Pharmacology and the rest of the Basic Science Departments. The other flight led downward into a basement apartment where my wife and I were to spend the next four years. Its major attribute was that it was within walking distance of the medical school, which meant that my wife could take the car each day to the elementary school at which she was to teach. But the entire apartment, consisting of a living-room, dining-room/kitchen, bath, and bedroom was about as large *in toto* as a respectable ordinary living-room. There followed four years of feet passing by the windows and dust sifting in from the St Louis air. The guts of the house were immediately next to us: the furnace, with its infernal network of pipes which led the steam heat throughout the building, a former 'mansion' which had been converted into apartments. Just across the hall from our apartment was one occupied by a medical student from an upper class who had also gone to my college in Mississippi. During the next couple of years, he was to perform the valuable function of keeping things in perspective for me since he had already undergone them. So living there had some merits—and the rent was cheap.

It was then that I put the figurative blinkers on, so as to keep my eyes pointing four years ahead. The first week of medical school was and is a blur. I do remember, while on my way to the school for the first day, meeting a young man named Syd Salmon; he was to become my anatomy lab partner and we have remained good friends over the ensuing years. There was a large auditorium in which the entire freshman class met. Of the remarks made by the Dean to the assembled group, which clearly represented all sections of the country and many major universities, I do not remember much. A most reassuring statement was made, however: 'We have picked the 85 best applicants from among hundreds of applicants across the country; we plan, in four years, to graduate that same 85.' The reassuring quality of that statement was to stand me in good stead many times throughout medical school. For such was not the case at all schools; one particular university in the South was notorious for 'flunking out' 15 per cent of the incoming freshman class.

Meanwhile, and a big 'meanwhile' it was to be, my wife began her daily four-year long series of drives to the elementary school, coping with snow, rain, reluctantly-educated children, and many hours of grading papers in the next room while I worked in anatomy. She was our only, and certainly our only visible, means of support. For my part, I was off to the anatomy laboratory. Off and running, *not* to coin a phrase.

For most freshman medical students, it is anticipation of the anatomy laboratory and its secrets that brings about the greatest fear and principal trembling. There is a graffito which I recall having seen etched in the sidewalk: *Gross Anatomy Really Is*. The laboratory was up the stairs and to the left through double doors with frosted glass, then through a veritable tunnel of display cases containing demonstration-dissections of different parts of the body. In the gallery of the room, there were about 45 or 50 marble-topped dissection tables, draped with canvas and concealing what clearly were ominously humanoid forms. The Professor of Anatomy was Dr Mildred Trotter, a woman in her sixties, slight, with completely white hair, and a gentle tone of voice. She explained in the class meeting the rules of the laboratory and how to begin and then we began—on the lower extremity. Syd, my laboratory partner, and I shared a cadaver, each working simultaneously on his 'half' of the body. The first task was to remove the outer skin so as to investigate the muscular and neurovascular structures of the leg. The leg is not complicated, certainly when compared with other areas of the body; it was for this reason that we began there. We used, most of us, small knives that required sharpening on a whet-stone periodically. Syd, however, chose for his dissection, what could only be described as a miniature machete: as I remember it, the blade itself was an inch and a half long and glittered as he worked. We were, as it turned out, of opposite temperaments in terms of the anatomy lab. Syd worked quickly, identifying the structures as we proceeded at our own paces. I worked meticulously, taking what I hoped was a careful and more surgical approach. We were therefore, Syd and I, often at different 'stages' in dissection. Syd finished the front of the leg before I did. The next portion of dissection was the back of the leg, which Syd decided to begin one Saturday afternoon, after class hours and without my knowledge. He made a tactical error which, in retrospect, he and I have laughed at many times: in order to approach the back of the leg, he simply turned the cadaver over and began to dissect. He forgot, however, to change sides of the table and it was therefore the back of 'my' leg on which he was operating! I realized this on Monday morning, to my chagrin; his apologies to me were profuse and were accepted as gracefully as possible.

Some in our class came to feel that anatomy lab was analogous to rolling the stone from the mouth of the cave daily, the cave from which the body was to have risen, but hadn't. For my part, I gloried in anatomy. The dissection of the hand, for example, that miraculous instrument. And it *was* miraculous to watch it emerging from its skin with all its intricacies, small muscles, and the long white tendons leading from the forearm out to the fingers to make them do the things of which only they are capable. It was luck and being in the right surgical plane that made my dissection happen to come out right. I remember Dr Trotter's approving look as she came to look at my work and found that it exhibited several points which she then demonstrated to the rest of the class. She took a small syringe and injected water into the tendon spaces and filled them as they might be in life and one could almost see the tendons slipping in their sheaths. I was very proud that morning. It was luck; but I felt like Leonardo.

The body on which we worked was that of a muscular athletic-appearing man in his fifties. The cause of his death was not at all apparent—until we entered the chest. There, on the aorta, the large vessel which leads outward from the heart and transports arterial blood to all sections of the body, was a large bulging aneurysm, which could have come only as a result of syphilis contracted years or decades before.

During the months before the discovery of the aneurysm and our sure knowledge that the cadaver had had syphilis, we could only conjecture about the cause of his death; his body became for us simply an object of scientific concentration and daily work. With our discovery, he suddenly became human again; our earlier concerns about anatomy laboratory flashed back in on us; this body *was* a man who had walked, talked, received and sent messages with his nervous system and made love with a woman who was, symbolically at least, still there on the table with him after all those intervening years. Ten years later, I succeeded in writing a poem about it.

It was also in anatomy lab that we began to make clinical correlations. Dr Cecil Charles, a practising physician with a PhD in Anatomy as well, often oversaw our work. I remember distinctly looking at the trigeminal nerve with him one morning and having him discuss with Syd and with me one clinical counterpart of that anatomical structure: a painful affliction consisting of excruciating stabs in one portion of the face along the distribution of the nerve and hence called trigeminal neuralgia—or as Dr Charles called it, Tic Douloureux (pronounced *Tick Dole-ah-roo*). The name still rolls off my tongue with pleasure.

Dr Trotter was of special help to me. She was always available to the students, always supportive. It was especially because I was doing well in anatomy that I went to her to discuss the fact that I was having difficulty with biochemistry, a course in the complicated chemistry of the body which I was taking simultaneously with anatomy. She received me most graciously in her office and listened while I expressed to her my concern. She said two things to me which in essence were as follows: You're doing a good job in Anatomy; don't let your other work suffer simply because you're having trouble in one area. She also said that she could not prescribe that advice for me had she not been in a similar predicament herself at times in the past. If she, now a brilliant professor, had in fact, *not* had such difficulties, she told a beautiful and necessary lie. Her support of my efforts, early in the freshman year, were absolutely pivotal to my subsequent successful completion of the year.

Of course there were other studies besides anatomy and I enjoyed all of them except biochemistry. I believe, in retrospect, I would have enjoyed that course as well because there were many dedicated teachers there (including Dr Carl Cori, who, with his wife, had won the Nobel Prize some years before). The fact is that the biochemistry course for the freshman class that year was being overseen by a young PhD, a man who in my conference with him seemed to have little or no concern with my problems at grasping the material and whom I would best characterize as simply a prig. Certainly he was no teacher. His basic lack of empathy for students and his apparently uncaring, abrupt manner with me has influenced me toward the opposite direction many times in my subsequent years as professor in a medical school.

The other courses during the freshman year went by rapidly and, except for the great amount of material presented to us, with relatively little difficulty. They included, for example, neuroanatomy and physiology, and microbiology, among others. But the first year was coming rapidly to a close. I remember two further outstanding incidents which have influenced me subsequently. In one lab, still using the partner system, one of the partners was to insert a rubber tube through the nose of his partner and into the stomach to retrieve gastric juice. The recipient of the tube was chosen by the flip of a coin and I lost. I'm afraid that I took it rather badly and with great difficulty, tears running down my cheeks from the discomfort. I have never since inserted a tube into a patient without a careful explanation of why it is necessary that it be done and simultaneously with the gentlest possible technique. Finally, when we studied the pelvis in anatomy, we learned that it is a very complicated structure in itself, its unique musculature and organs defying even the most careful first dissection. In a class on the female pelvis, Dr Trotter was working in her usual intense manner to have us understand the relations of one structure to another. She was trying particularly hard to have us understand that the walls of the vagina are, anatomically, usually in a state of collapse and apposition with one another. She followed this discussion with a simple statement, 'The vagina is a potential space.' A potential space, indeed. The phrase has stuck in my head for many years.

When the first year ended, I elected, rather than stay in St Louis for the summer doing research with one of the professors, to go to North Carolina with a friend in another medical school to try to make money toward next year's tuition. The method of making money seems, in retrospect, so ridiculous and full of folly, as indeed it turned out to be, that it seems worthy of a paragraph. We elected to sell Bibles in North Carolina, calling on the potential customers on a door-to-door basis and offering a selection of books, especially the very large family-type Bibles so popular among families in the South, at least in the past. The most popular type of Bible was about 15 inches wide, 20 inches tall, 5 inches thick, weighing about 8 pounds. It contained a central section in which the family tree could be written out and was clearly meant to be passed on from generation to generation. The same book could also be ordered with gilt edged pages, which looked very nice on the coffee table, for only three dollars more: $29.95. As I moved from door to door that summer, I couldn't help but think that many of the people on whom I called needed food and clothing more than a Bible. I suffered financially because of it, making only barely enough money to cover the cost of maintaining an apartment in St Louis as well as the expenses incidental to being in North Carolina. Many days, on rising, I gazed out the window and read whatever heavenly signs there happened to be as indicating I should definitely *not* go to work that day. But it was a great relief to be away from medical school for a three-month period and to come back to the second year, which was clearly to be more 'clinical'—as sophomores we were to meet our first real live patient—and to encounter our first fresh dead one.

September and the second year came inexorably. We returned to St Louis and to the basement apartment. And also to three of the courses which I remember most vividly: Pharmacology (study of the drugs used in medicine); Pathology (study of the process of disease, both grossly and microscopically); and Clinical Medicine, a series of lectures designed to introduce us to the clinical sphere, including interviewing of patients and physical examination. Pharmacology was a pleasure because we knew we were studying drugs which we would be using for the rest of our lives. Pathology offered us the contrast between the normal anatomy, which we had already studied, and the disease processes to which the body is heir.

It was in Pathology that I saw my first post-mortem examination: the examination of an infant who had died shortly after being born quite prematurely. While the professor explained to us the procedure of post-mortem examination, the several students gathered there looked on with wonder at the recently alive tissue. I questioned the professor silently and then aloud as to the exact reasons why such an infant, so small and yet so otherwise perfectly formed, had not lived. The professor's only answer was 'prematurity'. The word meant much more to him than it did to us: immature lungs, immature heart and nervous system, immature liver. But it still seems, even at this point, an inadequate explanation for such a tragedy.

There were slides, slides, and more slides. Slides flashed on a screen during what seemed to be hundreds of lectures; slides of every tissue and all the major diseases of those tissues about which we were to hear, then to read, then later to see. It was an exciting time because we could see that clinical medicine, although still off in the distance, was certainly closer than a year ago. In Clinical Pathology, we learned the systematic examination of blood and urine, and of every other body fluid. We examined each other's fluids. We learned, for the first time, to draw blood from each other. We learned, in short, what is *normal* for a hundred or more tests of every type and description. We thought it very difficult at the time. It turns out, of course, that *learning what is normal* is the hardest part of what every doctor has to do.

And we began to learn the art and science of physical

examination on each other through a series of lectures given in the spring. Each didactic session was followed by a 'practical' session during which we met in groups (of the same sex) to practise on each other the techniques of examination just covered. All this, of course, was in preparation for our first actual confrontation with a patient, which was to take place near the end of the second year. I remember especially how difficult it was to learn how properly to use the ophthalmo-scope, the instrument with the bright light which is used to examine the back of the eye; the procedure, once learned, is not difficult, but it requires concentration on the part of the physician and the patient in order that the light may pass through the dark diameter of the pupil and flash on the back of the eye where the blood vessels and the head of the optic nerve shimmer and finally focus like a chandelier.

I especially looked forward to acquiring my own stethoscope and purchased a very good one in spite of the fact that cheaper models were available: I felt, even at that time, the lure of the heart and its virtually ceaseless activity. I remember with great pleasure discovering that there was much more to the heart sounds than a simple 'lup-dup'—that there were splits in the sounds and noises made by the heart which, if carefully listened to, could lead to seemingly incredible feats of clinical diagnosis without the use of other tools. It was only last year, sixteen years after my first purchase of that stethoscope, that I finally turned it in for a new one, though of the same make and model.

We were required to purchase white pants and coats, other instruments, and a bag to carry them in for our first meeting with the patient, which was to be done in pairs. The requisite photograph of us, taken, of course, for 'posterity', shows us glaringly resplendent in our white coats, holding black leather bags and smiling. A series of examinations was done on Saturday mornings, two of us seeing the same patient, one taking a history of the patient's illness, and the other per-forming a physical examination. Our findings were then analyzed by a faculty member in some detail. It was our first encounter with a *lup-dup* that might be significant; with a liver that was clearly enlarged; and indeed with the laying on of hands.

If we looked almost like doctors, we fooled no one, neither the patients nor ourselves. We were encouraged to introduce ourselves to the patients as 'Doctor Blank', but the patients knew we weren't physicians, almost from the very first. At this point, we were simply learning to accumulate 'data' about the patients; the actual synthesis or clinical diagnosis was a long way off for us, a fact which quickly became apparent. We were as slow as turtles and sometimes laughingly inept: I remember my partner thumping like thunder on the *back* of one patient's chest while I was trying to listen to the *front*.

The word 'grateful' doesn't have exactly the right shade of meaning, but will have to do instead of the word, whatever it is, that would serve to say precisely how I feel now about those first patients. They gave themselves to us and we accepted them.

The last two years of medical school were almost purely 'clinical', as opposed to the first two which were 'basic science', in the main, and served to prepare us for what we would see in the hospital.

During the clinical years, we first began to 'live' in the hospital. Long hours were required, not only because we were learning, of course, but because the patients came in at all hours, and for the first time our efforts came to be really useful in their care. Being useful meant staying up all night, at times, but it was at these times that we seemed to learn the most. Basically, though, we were still ignorant: ignorant of the diagnostic skills which we saw displayed all around us by the interns and residents, people who *really were* doctors. We stood in awe of all the clinical facts that they had at their disposal.

'Rounds' is, I suppose, a curiously descriptive term, usually used to mean 'the professor' seeing, in turn, a group of patients with a group of students. It was during rounds that we first learned what clinical skill really means, how to handle difficult moments with a patient; in short, how it *should* be done. Dr Carl Moore, Chairman of the Department of Internal Medicine, served us as a perfect professor to emulate. One young woman, about my age and terribly ill with cystic fibrosis, a respiratory ailment sure to be fatal, stands out in my memory of rounds with Dr Moore. He took a careful history from the girl, performed an exemplary physical examination, all the while keeping the patient completely at ease. Afterwards, as the group of us, students and Dr Moore, turned to go, Dr Moore called our attention to a vase of flowers on the patient's bedside table. 'Someone must love you very much,' he said, 'to send you those beautiful flowers.' I realized, in that instant, that such a sensitive comment from a physician can be an absolutely vital part of whatever healing there is to be done.

Basically, the students 'rotated' in small groups every month or so on different clinical services: we became cardiologists for a month, then paediatricians, then neurosurgeons, orthopaedists, and all the rest. I liked Psychiatry very much, but I became gradually convinced that it would be too easy to take all my patients' problems home with me and reluctantly ruled out Psychiatry as a potential career.

I enjoyed Obstetrics. At Homer G. Phillips Hospital, I delivered over 30 babies and fell temporarily in love with some of the patients. It is easy to see how the great masters of painting often chose pregnant women for their subjects: they were so beautiful, in spite of their pain, and in spite of the absurd posture birthing requires. Delivering a child during a normal birth process is, of course, relatively easy for the doctor. But for a junior medical student, it was a profoundly moving experience during which I felt honoured to be a participant.

On Orthopaedics, I spent hours looking through a microscope for the bacillus that causes tuberculosis (but is difficult to find, at times, microscopically). I felt chagrined when the technician in the bacteriology lab found the slender red rods of TB easily, the first time. I only hoped that, in my prolonged contact with the patient, I hadn't breathed into my own lungs that bacillus, at the name of which I still think reflexly of poor John Keats. In fact, my skin test for TB did become positive during medical school, a finding which could only mean that I had, indeed, been exposed to the germ.

There were vast amounts of material to assimilate during each new rotation period. Jay Smith, Jerry Bauman and I often rotated together—and just before a test, the three of us usually got together to go over the material. With these two, studying was always fun: there was a sense of camaraderie like that at the foot of a mountain just before a climb. Each of us contributed his own bits of knowledge to the pre-test discussion. Jay was a 'list' man—bright and very organized in his approaches to studying. It used to worry me that he could list 'twenty causes of hypercalcemia' and I could never remember more than fifteen. He seemed to have lists for every question I might ask him. Jerry was logical, tenacious, and also bright. He, too, was more organized, I'm afraid, than I was. Just before the Parasitology exam, for example, he unrolled a giant sheet of brown wrapping paper; it was completely covered with lists of parasites, signs and symptoms, laboratory findings, and therapy: I was flabbergasted. Since each of us was married, our in-hospital work and study soon spilled over into whatever time there was for social gatherings. To say that we became close friends is still to understate the relationships that developed and persist to the present. I can still recall some of Jay's 'lists', but this time with amusement.

It became gradually clearer that Internal Medicine was the discipline for me; and within Internal Medicine, Cardiology was especially appealing. It seemed to me at the time, and still seems, that there is a logic to the way the heart works that is missing in some of the other disciplines. At any rate, it was easy for me and I resolved to learn all that I could about it. On my elective periods, and during the summers, I helped in cardiac research, listened to patients' hearts, looked at X-rays of hearts, and immersed myself in pure joy.

In the senior years, the medical student learns at which hospital he is to begin the post-graduate phase of his education, a phase which ranges in duration from one to five years and begins with that awesome first year of full patient-care responsibility, the Internship. For the first time, during our senior year, a computer was used to match the students with the hospitals (each ranking the other in order of their preference).

It was morning; there was an envelope and, inside the envelope, a computer card which read: Internship—Medicine; Strong Memorial Hospital/University of Rochester School of Medicine, New York. I was elated to be 'matched' at such a prestigious institution. My education in medicine had only begun: I was to spend five more years in post-graduate training in Medicine and Cardiology.

Today, at the medical school and hospital at which I teach and see patients, a brand-new intern told me the following story. While climbing a flight of stairs after the first full day of his internship, he met on the landing, coming down, an elderly man, bent and with a cane, but with the predictable shiningly alert eyes. The old man asked, 'Are you an intern?' On hearing the young doctor's tired, 'Yes', the old man followed up with another question: 'Do you know what it takes to be a good intern?' 'No sir, I don't.' 'Well, it takes the heart of a lion, the eye of an eagle, and the hand of a lady.'

Whether or not the phrase is original to the old man, his words give shape to a place in time that is true enough—and as good a place as any to stop. Or to begin.

Lesley Isenberg

Lesley Isenberg, the daughter of a London GP, was born in London in 1951. She was educated at Tottenham County School, and at the Welsh National School of Medicine, qualifying in 1974. Paediatrics and a rotation at the Whittington Hospital, London, followed house jobs, and she has just returned from working as a general practitioner locum in Australia.

To begin at the end of the beginning. Two weeks after qualifying as a doctor I arrived at a hospital in New-port, a bright green housewoman, pockets bulging with goodies and a head with sterile facts. In the first bed on the left in the male ward to which I was assigned, was a young man, who, hearing me push open the flap doors sat up, stared at me and then growled ferociously.

'Is he often like this?' I asked the gentleman in the next bed who had laid aside his *Sun* open at page 3.

"Im? Oh, 'e goes like that now and then. Leave 'im alone . . . 'e'll be alright. Needs 'is 'ead examined if you ask me.'

I looked back at the young man with grave misgivings. He lurched in a zig-zag fashion across his bed on all fours, dripping sweat and snapping in my direction. At the sound of his most turbulent howl yet, the ward Sister appeared before us.

'Good God,' she said. 'Mr Evan's gone hypo again.' And then, to me, 'Go and get some glucose, *sugar*'—the last word emphasized as if, with my newly-acquired qualification I had been enrolled in the book of idiots. Knowing the physiology, signs and symptoms of the state of a patient with a low blood sugar had not helped me recognize the simple cause of the young man's transformation into one of the larger cats. My medical schooling, it seemed was to continue beyond medical school . . . ad infinitum.

It had begun at the Welsh National School of Medicine five years prior to this embarrassing scene. Deciding upon medicine as a career had been difficult. Until the age of ten I had been attracted by telescopes and heavenly bodies. As a precocious Galileo I had already discovered the tenth planet and had revealed the secrets of the Martian canals. In my second decade I returned to earthly matters and decided to be an archaeologist. Joining a caravan trail across the little known Gunga Din wilderness I would achieve fame by chancing on the lean remains of a hitherto unknown civilization. One profession I would never consider was Medicine. Never!

All of which goes no way towards explaining how it was that in 1969, aged seventeen, I crossed the Severn Bridge and the English border into Wales, into Cardiff and into Medicine.

I think it was the supper-time conversations that did it. Nightly, the dramas of the dissection room and twitching frogs were enacted in the kitchen as my brother, then a first-year medical student in London, recounted the day's activities to the rest of the family. In a distinctly medical milieu I was steeped in the tradition of stories about missed diagnoses, narratives about the brilliant interpretation of a skin rash hitherto thought to be a benign spot. Up to the last minute I scoffed at all this but musing one night on the awful prospect of three years of studying zoology and psychology at university —a date for an interview at a northern university had arrived that morning in the post—I suddenly knew with most uncharacteristic certainty that I was hooked on the medical anecdote and had never really wanted to be au fait with the mating habits of the fruit fly Drosophila.

I ran next door to tell my brother of the dramatic turn in my life. With fraternal foresight he predicted a change of heart in the morning and turned to sleep. My heart, however, did not change. I wanted to be part of their world and I have no doubt that had my family been greengrocers or county cricketers I would have ended my days among the cabbages or in the slips rather than in the surgery.

With excitement I reapplied to UCCA for Medicine and listed the lucky six medical schools of my choice. With deference to my zoology teacher, Mr Davies, I included Cardiff. He told me it was a clean city. With such a recommendation what could I do but put it down . . . last on the list. Although keen to leave London it was a surprise even to me that, as a result of the twists and turns of applications, 'A' levels, interviews and fate, I landed at the Welsh National School of Medicine, Cardiff. It sounded like the other end of the earth.

In those days before the M4, when my parents took me down, it was a five-hour car journey. We saw the Wiltshire White Horse gazing across the hills; watched the Malborough boys pacing their town, sailed through Chippenham and sighted the Severn Bridge loping across the estuary. Later, I loved travelling by train to Cardiff. Most of all I liked the Sunday evening journey from Paddington. Always a good conversation could be had with a returning Welshman or a Swansea student wrapped in a green scarf. It was packed with travellers stolidly nourishing themselves with door-step sandwiches and Welsh cakes on the teetotal, slothful Sunday train. Past the evil lights of Llanwern steel works—the blue xenon piercing the black sky with uncanny automation; then the river of Newport, heavy and grand, its bends accentuated by the spiralling estates on the hillsides. Newport, twenty minutes to go . . . pick up bags, guitar, typewriter, cushions . . . and then Cardiff—a city of arcades and castles, long grey streets and corner shops, sad high skylines and rain. Hidden in the centre, near the museum and amongst red roads and cherry blossoms, lay the University buildings where I worked for the first two pre-clinical years.

As a constituent of the University of Wales, Cardiff Medical School had been in action since 1893. With my year, the intake of students took a giant leap in numbers from a compact seventy or so to 108. This coincided with the opening of the vast unfinished University Hospital of Wales at the Heath, overlooking the city. I was terrified at first. Imagine an inhabitant of the northern London suburbs, a virtual teetotaller, immensely ignorant, a short, stout and shy plodder being jettisoned into a cacophany of strangers. I retired, tongue-tied, to my Hall of Residence, increasingly miserable and despairing of ever feeling at home again. The rest of the year seemed so large and global, assured and knowledgable. About half were Welsh, some from the north. They sang and drank and played rugby loudly and seemed to know people in the years ahead of them in no time at all. There were about thirty girls, some of whom lived as I did during the first year, at an all female Hall of Residence in Penarth. Penarth is a tidy, stately seaside-town some six miles outside Cardiff. This was my pre-automobile era and so social life revolved around the last Cardiff to Penarth bus and the tea-tippling habits of the drivers. At first I felt so alien and alone but, gradually, I got to know people, mainly 'non-medics', and went debating, anti-apartheid demonstrating, singing and the like. For most of my pre-clinical years I saw little of my fellow-students outside working hours and it was not until the clinical years that I began to fit into the medical world.

Work divided into the three pre-clinical subjects: Physiology, Biochemistry and Anatomy. Within weeks we had slotted into a routine of lectures, tutorials, the occasional highlight of a clinical demonstration, and then more lectures. Physiology lived up to my expectations of being cruel to amphibians; and biochemistry seemed to consist of a stream of electron clouds and multivalent 'moles'. The practical sessions passed as happy hours of ineptitude. My biochemistry partner and I took the sessions with a pinch of salt . . . which may have been why most of the chemical recipes we tried failed to sulphate, bond, vaporize or in any way act as predicted in the manuals. And then Anatomy. My Lewis's *Grey's Anatomy* lay heavily on the desk at Penarth open at the most gory illustration. In theory I could see the attraction of poring over the minutiae of the relation of one viscus to another, but I hated dissection. The DR (Dissection Room)—a vast and sinister greenhouse growing waxen bodies in rows, was the object of my recurrent nightmares; yet the long hours of rote were at least lightened by the camaraderie of the dissecting team as we cheerfully chopped through vital structures, perforating a viscus or two whilst identifying incorrectly our gentleman's internal organs.

On one occasion we were taken on a tour of the department. Down in the embalming room lay a bloated virescent body on a cold slab complete with infusing tubes in strategic places. The room was cool, tiled and silent. Behind me I heard soft whispers in Welsh, followed by a cry. I turned to find a student slumped behind me. One down, one hundred and seven to go!

I regret to record the sad truth that for at least a year or two I was haunted by fallacious fancies of what I was missing by staying in Cardiff rather than being at Oxbridge or London. To Ros, a friend whose acquaintance I had made whilst admiring her histology sketches, I moaned endlessly about the lack of Cardiff's antiquity, lack of flowing gowns and punting on the Taff. With time and a growing circle of friends I tempered my demands and gradually began to enjoy myself. I moved into a flat by Roath Park with four non-medics. I went to 'Med Club', half learnt the Welsh National anthem and the 'Med Club' Medley and even saw a rugby match as part of my programme of assimilation into Celtic culture.

Suddenly, second MB—the great Slog—was upon us. My main worry was the anatomy viva. I had studied the mysteries of the bone with the aid of my trusty skeleton, sold to me in the early days by Mr P., the chief technician, who had assured me that with its four clavicles and three humeri it was indeed a fine specimen. Always bracketed with the Jones's for vivas, we of the middle alphabet were herded like greyhounds into traps for the starter's bell—at which we crossed the floor of the DR and met the examiners on the other side. There they sat, chuckling and twiddling the odd bone as they awaited their prey. I prayed not to be asked to identify a landmark on the living model: a technician press-ganged into stripping for the occasion. I wondered if he ever gave the game away . . .

'Down a bit . . . to the left . . . ask me to cough.' I knew that however obvious his deltoids or his clearly demarcated anatomical 'snuff box', there was no way, under stress, that I would identify them correctly. But no! They led me past this gentleman and on to a more recumbent and immobile fellow.

'Now, what do you call this, young lady?' The External Professor rocked on his heels, his kindly voice filtering through a nicotine-scarred larynx. He was pointing with his yellow fingers to a viscus in the lower reaches.

'Uterus,' I said, with no hesitation.

'Look again,' came the stern reply.

My heart plunged. Then I noticed an appendage, much altered by time and embalming fluid. There it was! Unless the poor chap had been a hermaphrodite the viscus had to be the bladder. Stammering, I rectified the mistake and saved myself from dismal failure by giving a Grant's Atlas account of the intrinsic muscles of the foot.

Being five foot short and a non-rugby player means that one does not see the pass list until almost everyone else has seen and digested it and whooped away. Finally, I saw my name on the list—but several of my friends' names were missing. The film of fatigue and uneasy dissatisfaction which always seems to come in the wake of exams came then. Later that week, having packed away all vestiges of anatomy books; sold my skeleton, four clavicles and all, to a first year student; sealed my physiology notes in a frog-proof strong box and moved my belongings into my next seat of residence—a mildewed mansion near the hospital—I was hit by a typhoon of elation half-way to London on the motorway. Two months of freedom! I was going to Italy and then to a job I had arranged as a cleaner in a local hospital. No more pre-clinicals! Real medicine at last!

They say the first two years are the worst. I knew things could only get better and they did. You may be relieved—as I was—to discover that I liked clinical medicine.

Mrs C. was my first patient. That is, she was the first lady clerked by L. Isenberg, Medical Student—First Year Clinical. A patient of the Metabolic Unit, she weighed twenty-one stone on entering the ward—and twenty-one on leaving! We were all disappointed. She had kept the other ladies and myself in hysterics by demonstrating how to make 100 calories of food look like a sumptuous repast by placing the plate in front of a magnifying shaving mirror and eating whilst looking at its reflection. With each mouthful of the giant food hologram she would wink at us and ripple with giggles.

The Metabolic Ward was the first to open in the vast, unfinished sprawl of the new University Hospital of Wales on the Heath. I was so disappointed to be sent there rather than to the older and more familiar hospital in town. Equipped with a replica of my father's stethoscope, a torch which actually worked, red and white hat pins and all the other paraphernalia of a clinical student in first flush, I was dying to work on a Florence Nightingale Ward with a hundred beds and central night light, plastered legs and bandaged heads. The Metabolic Ward was very sedate. Most of the patients' ills were not obvious to the untutored eye and with the crassness of the ill-informed, I felt cheated.

Having reached the first year clinical, we were then subjected to a horrendous timetable: we were guinea pigs in a new scheme of tuition. We were organized into three groups and rotated through six blocks of subjects over two years, the first-year clinical being put aside for endless introduction and other delaying tactics such as Pathology and Pharmacology. As practically all the hospitals in the Cardiff area were used by the students at various times, this necessitated a school bus to ship us around. The vehicle, termed the Wally Bus, was piloted by one Walter Stone, who would greet us after a long session in the wilds of Sully or Llandough, hands in pockets, pork pie hat set against the wind and a broad smile of welcome. He knew all the people in each year and could give us a run down on X's career or the names of Y's children and who was going to fail in the finals. His most telling remark, quoted in our 1974 Year Book was, 'I don't know what 'ave 'appened to people's brains.'

My brain, meanwhile, was busy trying to recall in what order to take a history, how to elicit reflexes, look at fundi and appear as if I had some inkling of what was normal hospital routine. I lived, at that time, in the very happy, mildewed house in Cosmeston Street. With four final-year Arts students as a willing audience I poured out the days' happenings and acted as their medical adviser on all manner of things from bunions to bilious attacks, giving as diagnoses whatever cases I had seen that day. In return for such inept advice I received instruction on Christopher Hill, Welsh history and F. R. Leavis. I appreciated their companionship greatly, suffered with them through finals and saw them off in June with the knowledge that this was the end of an era and that with my moving into a hostel at the Heath for the next year, I had finally become resident in the medical world.

On Friday nights—along with a companion or two—I would sometimes go along to Casualty at the Royal Infirmary and immerse myself in the real thing for an hour or two before returning to the rigors of studying Social Medicine and the 'Reorganization of the Health Service'. Basically, the 'real thing' consisted of my getting in everyone's way. Sometimes I did a bit of stitching, tried to put up an intravenous drip or take blood samples. The Consultant in Casualty took delight in showing us things: lumps, bumps, rashes—pointing out oddities of patients' speech and dress. I was listening to a conversation between him and a rather laconic registrar on the subject of the previous year's Christmas Show when a lady was wheeled in through the doors, the cold wind streaming in with her into the warmth. Her head was drooping onto her chest as she went past and I wandered into the cubicle in the wake of the Registrar to see some action.

I was shattered. I suppose she was the first acutely ill person I had ever seen. I thought she was dying. She was dying. She was choking, drowning in her own fluid; totally concentrating on her death. A little old lady, dank hair stuck around her head by cold sweat, every visible part moving in unison in her efforts to catch her breath. Her pale, clammy hands clutched the bars of the trolley, her eyes rolling upwards whilst her sounds were too near death to be heard. I wanted to run away . . . I had no idea what was wrong with her or what should be done. The Registrar quickly opened some vials on the side bench and injected their contents into a vein in her arm, taking a long time to do so. He fixed an oxygen mask to her nodding head, spoke a few words in a slow, unhurried way and beckoned me to follow him outside the cubicle. I accompanied him. What was it? What had he given her? Why was she dying?

'And then,' he said, leaning against the Casualty Officer's door, 'this physio comes on and does the dance of the seven veils . . .'

I was astounded. How could he stand around chatting whilst that lady lay only a few feet away? The answer was that, for him, this patient fitted into a well-known pattern. He had seen it before. He had recognized her heart failure, and treated it appropriately. Within half an hour we saw her recover enough to thank him and be wheeled off to the ward. I despaired of ever knowing enough to translate theory into practice. Medicine is all about patterns—the look of the old lady in heart failure, the way a sick child lies, the pain of peritonitis. It takes a lifetime to learn.

After months cooped up in tutorial rooms and libraries I eventually found myself walking, in the early hours of the morning, down the dim and narrow corridors of the Infirmary. My first surgical firm had its weekly emergency intake there and we stayed overnight on Thursdays to see red-hot appendices and highly-strangulated hernias and to keep the houseman company. Dogs and police cars in the Casualty yard at midnight; whisky at two am; letting retractors slip at vital moments, seeing the bleary dawn through the top windows of the theatre.

One night we were asked if someone would 'special' a lady

who might require surgery during the night for suspected abdominal trauma. The lady, a dashing redhead of at least seventy, had drunk herself to oblivion at a birthday party (not her own) and then floated down two flights of stairs, ending up pinned to the top of a bannister. Maybe her spleen had been torn? Somehow I found myself placed by her bedside, recording dials and mysterious fluid levels every fifteen minutes. In the still ward the light over her bed made great hollows of her eyes, hooded, smudged in purple eyeshadow, and ringed in tear- and trauma-proof mascara. Just as I was dropping off, her blood pressure nosed groundward, her fluid levels careered in the same direction and she was whisked off to the theatre.

A friend on the same firm came along with me to see the operation. We stood in the changing-room quite baffled by the range of theatre wear. We tried various combinations of baggy trousers, masks and those bits of pink paper whose purpose I have never understood. Should we take all our clothes off and then put on the baggy trousers or were they boiler suits to go on top of everything else? We peeped out of the changing-room hoping unsuccessfully to catch the eyes above a mask. We ventured out ready to retreat if challenged. I made the mistake of offering assistance to the Consultant Anaesthetist who, in standard baggy bottoms, looked just like the theatre technician.

The 'Respiratory' block is linked in my mind with winter, with Christmas, with dark afternoons and the deep moan of the steamers on the starboard side of Sully Hospital on Sea. Sometimes only two or three of our firm made it out there in the Wally bus through the still and frosted lanes of Penarth, but it was worth it if only to be taught by Dr Foreman, a chest physician on Sully's starboard side. He was at home and at ease with the coal-scarred miners and he talked simply and lucidly to them and to us. With good humour and gentleness he conducted us through the wards. I hope I shall always remember what he taught us from polyphonic noises, the problems of sick budgerigars and nicotine, all the way through to his bedside manner.

Around Christmas time of that year we staged the Hospital Christmas Show. Named from time immemorial 'Anencephalics' (a tribute no doubt to the detailed neuro-anatomy of the medical students who script and present it), it occupied the majority of my time for many months. I enjoyed it so much that from then on I dabbled in a variety of theatrical ventures at the Heath until old and crippled by Finals.

The next diversion on the agenda was the Elective Period. For three months we were at liberty to tramp the world and enjoy life provided that at the end of the period we returned armed with a serious tome expounding our medical experiences. I went to Zaria in Northern Nigeria. In that arid world I saw people with obvious ills, with the grossest pathology. I have a stream of pictures in my head of Zaria; the flat land broken by yellow inselbergs; yams and yet more yams; our bungalow; the children's emergency unit; the little boy with nephrotic syndrome who taught me to count in Hausa; the mental hospital in Kaduna . . . a thousand miles of drought.

I returned to the final year, eager to be finished, qualified and aiming for the East or perhaps Africa again.

I had moved for the last time and went to live at Howard Gardens, a small inbred community down by the Infirmary in town. Opposite us there was a bowling green where I sat one Sunday after another, reading about fractures and the multitudinous causes of joint pains. Occasionally we thought about finals, but life was relatively uninfluenced by that morbid event until after Christmas. My schedule was arranged so that right up to two weeks before finals I was engaged in the most strenuous and enveloping block of all—that dealing with obstetrics and paediatrics. For much of those three months I lived in at the hospital. There were only two of us on each firm. We shared a room at St David's, the maternity hospital, and divided up deliveries between us and the midwives. Then we spent hours at Llandough, waiting for gynaecological emergencies to come bleeding out of the night air, comforted by the

Llandough cherry pies topped with that splodge of artificial cream which made Llandough such a gastronomic centre.

I delivered seventeen babies and seemed to attract a special line in teenage single mothers who did not want their children, male or female. Then we moved on to paediatrics. We sat petrified in paediatric cardiology clinics knowing that our unforgivable ignorance would be found out sooner or later. Case conferences at the Heath, ward rounds in the special care baby-unit conducted in an ambient temperatuie of 90°C —it was a crowded time.

The Howard Gardens self-tutorial system for Finals broke down very quickly. We aimed to spend weekends tutoring each other on subjects we had read up that day. The discussion usually began in earnest but ended at Med Club or in the local pub. Months were going by so quickly. It was impossible to believe that very soon all this would end. Already we were applying for house jobs; some were marrying; all were planning and ready to disperse. How could I leave now that life had gained rhythm? I cursed finals and the end which they signified. Instead of applying for jobs in London as I had planned to do during the first two unhappy years, I aimed to stay in Wales for at least the houseman's year.

As the pace to finals quickened, so the ranks closed. Every available moment was occupied seeing rare endocrine abnormalities in the metabolic wards. We spent hours in the Cardiology wards desperately trying to distinguish third heart sounds from murmurs, clicks and late systolic whoops. Having shied away from the Coronary Care Unit when assigned to it for fear of the Sisters, catheters, monitors and exposed uncomfortable bodies, I now returned to study ECG's. I suddenly developed a mania for skin clinics and neurology demonstrations! Sometimes the hysteria in the kitchen at Howard Gardens was unbearable.

The final exams were not so awesome as in previous years, our continual assessment having accounted for some proportion of the marks already. However, that did not prevent my adrenalin levels reaching an all-time high as I waited to be called for the clinical section.

When it was all over I joined a party rowing on Roath Lake. The results were to be published some time that evening. We drifted around the lighthouse armed with wine, songs and impromptu renderings of speeches from Richard III. Just as, arriving at Cardiff, I had been fearful of the five years to come, so now I was again afraid. Here, within the banks of my student life I was in calm and secure waters. I did not want to see the pass list with its message of change, housejobs, and far-off countries. I was happy where I was.

About ten people told me I had passed before I saw the evidence for myself. It seemed like a giant hoax; surely it was a huge mistake? The Final Year Dinner was held a week later. Max Boyce, the guest artist, sang, 'We all had doctors' papers', to everyone's delight. I could see him through a myopic mist and crowds of familiar outlines less distant. Opposite me, a beaming and jocular consultant was telling a joke, his eyes creasing as he delivered the punch line in Welsh. Then, as he translated the nub of the story into English for my benefit, suddenly the transient nature of my five years at the Welsh National School of Medicine hit me full force. Somebody gave me a red rose, and lots of people said goodbye.